Occupational Therapy
Activities From Clay
To Computers
Theory And Practice

Occupational Therapy
Activities From Clay
To Computers
Theory And Practice

Estelle B. Breines, PhD, OTR, FAOTA
Clinical Associate Professor
Department of Occupational Therapy
New York University
New York, New York

 F. A. DAVIS COMPANY • Philadelphia

F. A. Davis Company
1915 Arch Street
Philadelphia, PA 19103

Printed in the United States of America

Last digit indicates print number: 10 9 8 7 6 5 4 3 2 1

Allied Health Editor: Lynn Borders Caldwell
Production Editor: Crystal S. McNichol
Cover Design By: Steven R. Morrone

As new scientific information becomes available through basic and clinical research, recommended treatments and therapies undergo changes. The author and publisher have done everything possible to make this book accurate, up to date, and in accord with accepted standards at the time of publication. The author, editors, and publisher are not responsible for errors or omissions or for consequences from application of the book, and make no warranty, expressed or implied, in regard to the contents of the book. Any practice described in this book should be applied by the reader in accordance with professional standards of care used in regard to the unique circumstances that may apply in each situation. The reader is advised always to check product information (package inserts) for changes and new information.

Library of Congress Cataloging-in-Publication Data

Breines, Estelle B.
   Occupational therapy activities from clay to computers : theory and practice / Estelle B. Breines.
     p.   cm.
   Includes bibliographical references and index.
   ISBN 0-8036-1145-5 (soft)
   1. Occupational therapy.   I. Title.
   RM735.B74 1995
   615.8′515—dc20
                                                  94-6968
                                                  CIP

To Sylvia Goldin Borgman Forman—who made my life and my work possible.

Other books and publications by the author:

Perception: Its Development and Recapitulation

Origins and Adaptations: A Philosophy of Practice

Functional Assessment Scale

Proprioceptive Schematic Orientation: A Mobilization Technique for the Upper Extremity, with Y. Ahmad, C. Lerke, and R. Reffler

Foreword

Dr. Estelle Breines is one of the true intellectual leaders in the field of occupational therapy. In this book, she has combined an analysis of the profession's intellectual history up to the present day with practical guidelines for the teaching and use of occupation as a therapeutic method. This is a major achievement.

This book spans a remarkable range of topics, from human evolution to the use of flat-nose pliers, from philosophy to beeswax (used in bookbinding), and from human development to computer power pads. Only an occupational therapist could have written this book! Our knowledge base is broad, and it is deep. It is esoteric, and it is eminently practical. Dr. Breines' book reflects the unique topical range of our profession.

Dr. Breines based this book on her years of experience in teaching entry-level occupational therapy students at New York University. This book is most effective in demonstrating that the profession of occupational therapy is a living, evolving entity with a fascinating past and an open-ended future. Entry-level students of occupational therapy need to understand this evolutionary quality of their new profession. There is a tendency for many new students to want to learn all the "facts" and "protocols" of "standard" occupational therapy practice. Sometimes entry-level students want a standardized set of terms and procedures reflecting "generally accepted" patterns of clinical reasoning. The evolutionary approach taken in this book is excellent in demonstrating to the student that the profession of occupational therapy is not a static, concrete entity with rigid definitions for every relevant phenomenon. Indeed, just as the profession has been able to accommodate different schools of thought in the past, so the profession will be able to accommodate unforeseen ideas in the future. The challenge to students is not to learn every technique of current practice but to take on a personal sense of responsibility for renewing the profession in the future. A profession's evolution is a creative act. To use Dr. Breines' terminology, the renewing of a profession is a wholesome occupation.

Like human evolution and the evolution of society, the evolution of a profession is not a random, totally plastic process. The profession of occupational therapy has evolved out of a set of organizing principles that are continuously rediscovered and reapplied in new social circumstances. The most important of these principles is the idea that occupation is a powerful force for human health. Dr. Breines' historical research on the intellectual roots of the profession of occupational therapy is as original and important as any other historical work done by a living author. Her special contribution to our knowledge of our own history is her documentation of the influences of the philosophy of pragmatism on early occupational therapy schools. Dr. Breines has shown how the ideas of John Dewey, probably the most influential proponent of pragmatism, influenced the curricula of early schools of occupational therapy and influenced the clinical reasoning of occupational therapy practitioners. John Dewey believed that occupation is a powerful force in human development and education. A reasonable generalization of that idea was that occupation could be a powerful force in restoring persons with disabilities to health and in preventing further disabilities. Hence, occupational therapy. Dr. Breines mapped out the person-to-person, event-to-event processes by which Dewey's ideas had their influences on the new profession. While recognizing that other ideas, such as moral treatment and the arts and crafts movement, also influenced the thinking of the founders, Dr. Breines has helped fill in and correct the overall historical picture. Such a correction can aid us in our future evolution.

Like Dewey's ideas on evolution, this book considers occupations from "clay to computers." Ancient occupations retain a place in our society, in this book, and in the practice of occupational therapy. However, to Dr. Breines' credit, this is not just a crafts book, and it does not just provide a way of analyzing occupations important to survival in the distant past. Occupations characteristic of industrialism are described. Photography, videotaping, computers, and telecommunications are analyzed as occupations of our age. Most important, the book recognizes that "the future is now" and that potentially therapeutic occupations are emerging at all times. Dr. Breines does not fear change and wishes to prepare students for theory and practice over long careers in an uncertain future.

Another useful feature of the book is its use of brief case studies that illustrate points with concrete examples of patients involved in occupations. Students will appreciate this feature of the book. This will help them see that the history and the theory do indeed have practical applications in promoting the health and well-being of real people. This will help them see that a profession is not just a set of techniques and that a professional is not just a well-trained technician.

In conclusion, I urge the students who read and use this book to study it well, the abstractions as well as the practical realities. These students are the future of our profession. I believe that Dr. Breines would join me in urging them to take active charge of that future. By building on the principles related in this book, our students are invited to go beyond us in scholarship and wisdom in creating the future evolution of our profession of occupational therapy.

David L. Nelson, PhD, OTR, FAOTA

Preface

Purposeful activity is the basis of occupational therapy. Yet, since the field began, occupational therapists and students have had many questions about this topic of such critical importance to the field. What is purposeful activity? Are the terms "activities," "crafts," and "purposeful activity," synonymous, or do they mean different things? Should crafts be used as therapy? What skills should therapists learn? Which media, modalities, and methods should be studied? Which should be used in practice? And when they are used, is it more important to do an activity or to do it well?

This text attempts to answer these questions by emphasizing how human activities originated and changed over time in a process called occupational genesis, and how this process contributed to learning, health, and survival of the human race. This book defines crafts and modern technologies as purposeful activities or occupations that contributed to the survival and development of humankind. Most important for occupational therapists, these human occupations are tools for therapy.

To structure an understanding of occupation, this text explores the relationships among the following:

1. Activities that have been used as clinical tools by occupational therapists from the inception of the field to today
2. The evolution of activities as survival tools for ancient peoples in the various roles they played in their societies and modern technology as an evolutionary extension of earlier activities
3. The value of old and new activities as learning tools in the developmental activities of children and adults as they aspire to assume their roles in society.

By examining relationships among people, their tools, their materials, and their societies, human development is viewed here according to the occupations in which people find meaning for their lives, from child to adult and from ancient to modern times. This relationship serves as the foundation for understanding occupational therapy's history and the profession's goal of bringing people to their highest level of functioning in their society, through the use of activities that are meaningful to the patient or client.

Making connections between these elements of human experience will give occupational therapy students and therapists the rationale, skill, and conviction to retain the useful tools of the past when they are pertinent and to reject them when they are not, as they keep up with society's newest inventions and adaptations. If this approach is successful, therapists will demonstrate confidently their right to use society's oldest and newest devices as therapeutic tools—infinitely—as humans continue to evolve and create.

Estelle B. Breines

Acknowledgments

Where does one begin to recognize those people who contribute to one's work, when that work represents a lifetime of learning? I guess, at the beginning.

My love for crafts and art began as a young child. When I was 4 years of age, Grandma Goldin, better known as Whitey, taught me to make a doll's dress from an old pillow case. I cut out the pattern, learned to thread the needle, and sewed the seams. I remember vividly how my doll fit into that coarsely made garment. When I was 5 and World War II erupted, my mom, Sylvia Borgman, began to knit for the sailors as if she were the sole provider of their clothing. I soon was stitching right along with her. I cannot remember learning to knit; I feel as if I always knew how. As the war progressed, Mom did the casting on, increasing, decreasing, and finishing. She let me work on the bodies of the sweaters. By age 8, we sat together in the movie theater knitting in the dark.

My dad, Sanford Borgman, taught me perspective and sparked my interest in perception and creativity. He was a fine artist who had won a scholarship to Cooper Union but chose instead to earn his living at pharmacy. His love of art was as contagious as his love for science. He took me to museums and to art classes, as his evening work hours gave us days together. I sat and drew for hours, but I never reached his level of skill. I became entranced with the many things one could make of materials and their roles in the lives of ancient and distant peoples.

When it was time to choose a career, occupational therapy was a natural. Here, I could combine my art and science interests. It was a time in the profession when, along with one's science studies, one learned to do every craft imaginable. I still have several treasures that I made in school.

The years passed, and I decided to write a book. Actually, I wrote a course. I was determined to show students the glories of activities and the brilliant thinking that established our profession on these ideas, and it seemed natural to develop a book to accompany the course. I am particularly grateful to Jane Miller, MA, OTR, who influenced me to begin this project and helped me with the early writing.

Eva Siegel, OTR, the laboratory instructor in our course, researched and designed a number of the activities. As one of my first fieldwork supervisors, it seemed fitting that we join in this classroom endeavor. Others who worked in the course over time are Priti Agarwal, OTS; Gloria Graham, MA, OTR; Laurell Jeffreys, OTR; Laura Lee Johnson, MA, OTS; Virginia Kim, MA, OTR; Marie Leo, MA, OTR; George McDermott, OTR; Betty Pang, OTR; Joanne Saggese, MA, OTR; Anna Soto, MA, OTR; and Irene Wilson, MA, OTR. Their ideas merged with mine and undoubtedly appear in this book, but they are not responsible for any errors; these are mine alone.

I also learned from the students. Some tested the instructions, some taught techniques, and some just asked good questions. Margo White, MA, OTR read an early draft and urged me on. Shari Grey, MA, OTR did illustrations. Mitchell Ehrlich, OTS wrote much of the video section, and Norman Askinazi, OTS did the activity analysis.

The following reviewers, who are all occupational therapy educators, deserve special recognition:

Sandra K. David, OTR/L
Senior Staff Therapist/Clinical Educator
Department of Occupational Therapy
Medical College of Georgia Hospitals and Clinics
Augusta, Georgia

Patricia M. Holz, OTR
Program Director and Instructor
Occupational Therapy Assistant Program
Fox Valley Technical College
Appleton, Wisconsin

Edith Carter Fenton, MS, OTR/L
Coordinator
Occupational Therapy Assistant Program
Becker College
Worcester, Massachusetts

Jacqueline L. Jones, PhD, OTR/L
Associate Professor and Chair
Department of Occupational Therapy
Elizabethtown College
Elizabethtown, Pennsylvania

Nancy Whiting Glover, MS, OTR/L
Program Head
Occupational Therapy Assistant Program
Stanly Community College
Albermarle, North Carolina

Ellen Berger Rainville, MS, OTR/L, FAOTA
Assistant Professor
Department of Occupational Therapy
Springfield College
Springfield, Massachusetts

Helene Goldstein, OTR/L
Assistant Professor
Department of Occupational Therapy
Creighton University
Omaha, Nebraska

Phyllis Barrett Samara, OTR/L, FAOTA
Professor of Occupational Therapy
Quinsigamond Community College
Worcester, Massachusetts

They taught me new methods, corrected my errors, made excellent suggestions about how to make this book more useful for students, and supported its publication. Without them this would be a pipe dream yet.

Other colleagues who offered suggestions, corrected my grammar, argued with me over concepts, and still stayed my friends are too numerous to mention. The ones who reviewed case examples and clinical comments and shared references, ideas, directions, and other good things are Claire Daffner, MA, OTR, FAOTA; Catherine Gordon, EdD, OTR; Deborah Labovitz, PhD, OTR, FAOTA; Elizabeth Lannigan, MA, OTR; Sharon Lefkofsky, PhD, OTR; Dina Loebl, EdD, OTR; Karen Macdonald, MA, OTR; Jane Miller, MA, OTR; and Elizabeth Torcivia, OTR.

My sincerest appreciation to the vendors who generously permitted the inclusion of photographs and illustrations: Tandy, Inc.; Fred Sammons, Inc.; American Art Clay Co., Inc.; S & S, Inc., and the NAMES Project, for the photograph of the AIDS memorial quilt.

Lynn Borders Caldwell of F. A. Davis Company saw the need for this book from the outset and never failed to give me her support. Her editorial comments made this text more readable, since I occasionally tend to write in tongues.

And yes, Ira, my blessed and tolerant helpmate, and the kids. Without them all, I could not have done it. Now recognize that the kids have kids, and yet they are all my kids; the ones that I bore, and the ones who came later. They helped in many different ways. Eric Breines contributed significantly to the computer and technology sections. Deborah Breines did most of the photography. Jacqueline Breines Danino, Esq., selected and organized the illustrations. Dr. Roxanne Breines Sukol guided the case example descriptions and assisted with certain aspects of the research. David and Alexsandra Breines and Talia and Eli Sukol tested activities with me. This book is as much a heritage for them and the younger grandchildren as anything.

Contents

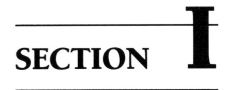

SECTION I

THEORY

1

Meaningful Activity

Human beings define their lives, cultures, values, and worth through activities. This principle is fundamental to occupational therapy. The history of human occupations from their origins to the present can tell us much about the meanings activities have for people. Understanding these meanings can guide therapists. This chapter discusses how occupations have evolved over the millennia. John Dewey, the great educational philosopher and pragmatist, adopted this model of social change as an educational tool to introduce meaning to his students by learning through activities.[1,2] These ideas about learning through doing were adopted by pioneers of our field and serve as foundational concepts for the profession.

GENESIS OF OCCUPATIONS

Over time, the nature of human activity has changed. Historians, anthropologists, sociologists, and others have studied these changes to understand their meaning. Two familiar patterns have been described. One explores the materials and tools people used during each age. The other reveals developments in the nature of work itself (Table 1-1).

The two parallel sequences shown in the table illustrate the relationships among people, their activities, tools, and materials from age to age. Approximate origins of these periods are indicated. Activities from each age are represented in modern society, and there are societies functional today that resemble each of these periods.

To illustrate how time has changed the relationships among these aspects of human occupation, the activities described in this book are organized along the lines of the evolutionary model of John Dewey, the world-re-

Table 1-1. EVOLUTION OF OCCUPATIONS FROM EARLIEST TO MODERN TIMES

Ages	Occupations
Stone Age (ca. 100,000+ BCE*)	Hunters and gatherers
Bronze Age (ca. 4000 BCE)	Nomads
Iron Age (ca. 250 CE†)	Farmers and artisans
Industrial Age (ca. 1700 CE)	Manufacturers
Technologic or Communication Age (ca. 1950 CE)	Communication technologists

*BCE—Before the common era.
†CE—Common era.

nowned educational philosopher, who is widely recognized for "learning through doing."[3] Dewey viewed human occupations in a historical perspective, and he used this approach as a teaching tool. For example, his students first learned about and performed the activities of peoples such as the North American Indians, and in doing so, learned skills relevant to their own lives. The students then learned the activities of agricultural societies such as the American pioneers, furthering their knowledge of society, literature, mathematics, and so on. The model of occupational genesis shows the relevance of activities for development and evolution, health, and human survival.

The ever-present genesis of occupations grounds the meaningfulness of activity. That is, activities develop to meet the needs of the present culture, and the relevance of the activities alters as time passes and needs change.

In essence, this approach is designed to (1) offer a rationale for past, present, and future activities that is consistent with occupational therapy philosophy and history; (2) produce respect for the kinds of activities that were meaningful in the past but are sometimes undervalued in modern times; and (3) prepare therapists to greet new and future activities with appreciation and confidence.

TOOLS FOR PRACTICE

Starting with the crafts of early peoples, this book follows a path that leads through tasks of the industrial and technologic revolutions as we currently know them, using electricity and communications media, and goes on to future activities we can only anticipate. This path illustrates how human beings develop new ways of dealing with the world around them. This book does not contain a comprehensive collection of activities. Rather, a range of simple tasks has been gathered from among the many activities human beings have devised during their time here on earth. These tasks represent the diverse activities found in one form or another in many cultures throughout the world and throughout the ages.

Many of these same activities, like the baskets and pots of ancient peoples, are traditional practice tools; some like photography are more recent and are characterized as technology. In all cases, they have been used in clinical practice at one time or another and are useful to therapists today as they adapt this knowledge in ways that can alter the functioning of minds and bodies in positive directions.

Because changes in the world and its activities are taking place at staggering speed, this documentation itself is becoming obsolete. Ideas are illustrated here to enlighten the beginner and to strike a thought in the minds of those who are experienced and particularly to show that activities evolve according to the meaning they have for human beings and that this relevance must be taken into consideration in the clinical environment. For activities to be therapeutic they must be meaningful, and meaningfulness is determined largely by the culture in which one lives.

Therapists need a broad array of skills to meet the needs and interests of their patients. Yet, understanding the origins of these beliefs and knowing how to use crafts and technology as tools for health does not assure the meaningfulness of these activities to patients. Providing meaning to patients requires other skills and perspectives.

Students must become adept at manual and technologic skills so that they can use them as therapy, and they must become skillful in determining when use of these activities is not therapeutic. Thrusting activities on patients is not therapeutic when those activities are not relevant to the patients' lives. Consequently, a therapist's repertoire must span a broad range to meet the widest variety of patients' needs and interests, regardless of diagnosis or functional deficit. Both manual and technologic skills are the profession's tools of practice; both are essential elements of human endeavor. If students and therapists expect to be prepared to meet patients' needs in this modern era, they must become proficient in activities of all sorts.

FINDING MEANING IN ACTIVITIES

Patients and therapists can find meaning among all of these activities, whether focusing on their survival role, their role in artistry, or their therapeutic value. If a task has meaning for an individual, it has purpose and merits use. That is, it is purposeful for that individual. The therapist's job is to find that meaning for patients while leading them through the therapeutic process.

For many patients, craft activities can be meaningful even if they are not self-care tools in the sense that our ancestors understood them. Today, there is a resurgence of the use of natural materials as art forms, making it easier to illustrate that craft art is valuable and that making objects is satisfying (Fig. 1–1). However, taking this idea into the clinic requires skill on the part of the therapist, both in presentation and in craftsmanship. Even mundane items need to be made skillfully for patients to regard them with respect.

Remembering the crafts one did as a child can elicit positive or negative feelings. Even if those memories are pleasant, producing childish objects does not create self-respect in adults. Such activities certainly will not be appreciated by those who learned from experience to belittle crafts. Therefore, not all patients will benefit from making handcrafted objects. Products need to be of a quality and design that the patient and others will value, aside from other therapeutic implications. Feelings of competence depend on positive feedback from others and are critical to the therapeutic process.[4] Well-crafted objects garner respect. Junk does not. Therefore, activities must be selected with skill. Choosing tasks at which patients can be successful will allow them to produce a quality product that will grant self-respect as well as respect from others.

Competence is not an issue for patients alone. Students and therapists must become competent in a range of skills if they intend to demonstrate them to others, develop confidence in their own abilities, and gather respect for those abilities.

Patients are often attracted to familiar activities. However, newly acquired disabilities can prevent patients from performing up to former standards. Therefore, using familiar tasks as therapy can highlight patients' dysfunctions, when just the opposite should be occurring. Sometimes teaching new activities can be a better

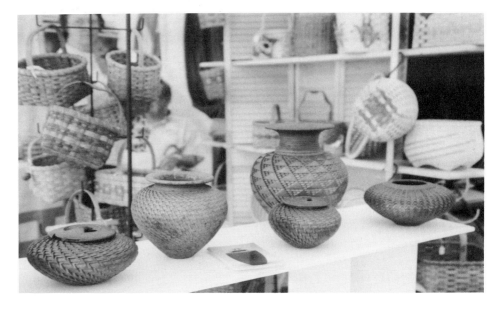

Figure 1–1. Clay pots in the foreground resemble the woven baskets displayed behind them. (Craft Fair, Peters Valley, NJ, 1993.)

way to develop skills. Old or new, familiar or unfamiliar, all activities have potential for healing the mind and the body. Selection of activities should emerge from collaborative decision-making between patient and therapist, toward therapeutic ends.

Some activities are too demanding for patients to complete. Effective activity analysis enables the therapist to identify parts of activities that patients can accomplish so that they can feel as if they are valuable participants in a larger task. In this way, groups can work together on activities, or individuals can work apart from one another to complete the many parts of a single job.

Contributing to a task that is larger than one can complete alone can be meaningful beyond measure, as

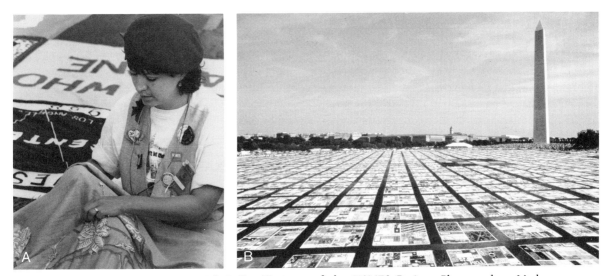

Figure 1–2. AIDS Memorial Quilt. (Courtesy of the NAMES Project. Photographer, Mark Theissen.)

long as one values one's contribution to the larger effort. One of the reasons that weaving is rarely seen in the clinic any longer, although it used to be widely used, is that as the length of hospital stays is reduced, few patients have the time to complete a whole project themselves, and no larger goal for the project has meaning for them. Yet, establishing a goal often engages people in efforts larger than they can accomplish on their own. For example, the AIDS memorial project that has been under construction since the mid-1980s has been meaningful to the extent that extraordinary numbers of individuals contributed embroidered and appliquéd segments to a mammoth craft project that drew strangers together in a common effort (Fig. 1–2).

OCCUPATIONAL THERAPY IDENTITY

Despite their convictions about the value of purposeful activity, therapists' questions about their practice re-emerge time and time again. These questions about practice and education can be found in generations of occupational therapy literature, some reaching back to the founding of the profession. In reality, the questions therapists raise about their practice and their beliefs are of such importance that the answers establish the profession's identity. Yet, its identity is precisely what occupational therapists have repeatedly sought to define.

Occupational therapists' uncertainty about their profession is reflected in the uncertainty of others. Before others can have a clear understanding of occupational therapy, the profession must answer its own questions —for without their resolution, therapists' certainty and confidence are jeopardized, preventing their patients from being served with the effectiveness they are due. Without confidence in the value of activity as therapy, patients will be hard pressed to understand the meaningfulness of occupational therapy for their own health and well-being.

Knowing that occupational therapists come from a heritage of great intellectual strength founded in theories of adaptation, evolution, development, and learning can make it clear that their training prepares them for changes in the modern world. Once therapists under-

stand their origins, they will be able to answer questions about the profession with certainty. By understanding their beginnings, therapists will be better prepared to make the decisions necessary for the healthy growth of their profession and for the welfare of those with whom they work. In addition, they will be ready to apply their skills without hesitation—while they and the world, their tools, and their activities continue to adapt and grow.

OCCUPATIONAL GENESIS AND OCCUPATIONAL THERAPY

The process of growth and connection among activities of the past, present, and future is termed "occupational genesis." Occupational genesis describes the evolving adaptive process in which humans engage in purposeful activities that are meaningful to their lives as their world and their experiences change. Occupational genesis emphasizes the expanding productivity of human beings as they engage in meaningful adaptive living throughout their lives.

Occupational genesis also details how these changes occur within each lifetime. In all societies, the activities of children prepare them for their roles as responsible adults. Skills developed in childhood continue developing throughout life in healthy individuals. Skill development is not only a feature of learning but is also a feature of health (Fig. 1–3).

Occupational therapists adopted these developmental and evolutional concepts as their traditional tools of practice because they offer meaning to patients' lives. Adaptation and grading of activity, both evolutional themes, are applied in all areas of practice using meaningful, purposeful activities to develop skill in all areas of function. Occupational therapy is a viable profession based on a firm, yet malleable foundation: the concept of adaptation and evolution. As long as occupational therapy remains open to the new directions society takes, we can be certain it will move easily and with health into the future, gaining strength as it gains history.

To develop these ideas, the genesis of occupations will be further explored from their origins in prehistory into

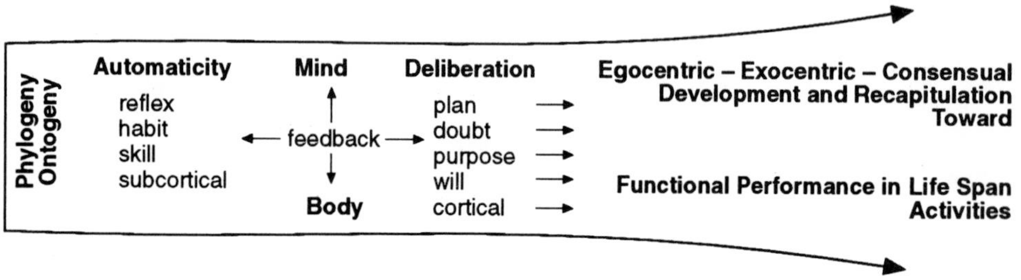

Figure 1–3. Model of Occupational Genesis. (From Breines, EB: Genesis of occupation: A philosophical model for therapy and theory. Australian Occup Ther J 37:47, 1990, with permission.)

the modern era. Ancient activities are correlated with those of modern civilization. Crafts and technology are shown to be meaningful activities, whether used for play or work, artistry or function, self-care, or the care of others.

Despite differences in materials, tools, and tasks, ancient and modern work skills have served the same survival needs for human beings. In turn, the skills of survival become creative arts. This merging of creativity and active occupation will be examined to learn the meaning of activity for human existence and health.

In summary, this book has been written to be used as a source book, not a cookbook, for there are no hard-and-fast solutions to human problems; each individual is unique, with a unique set of interests, abilities, and obligations that dictate meaning to life. It is hoped that creative therapists will adapt these ideas, expanding their repertoires beyond the limits of these pages, in keeping with the unique needs of their patients and their own special interests and expertise, offering meaning to each of their lives.

REFERENCES

1. Breines, EB: Origins and Adaptations: A Philosophy of Practice. Geri-Rehab, Lebanon, NJ, 1986.
2. Mayhew, KC and Edwards, AC: The Dewey School: The Lab School of the University of Chicago, 1896–1903. Appleton-Century, New York, 1936.
3. Ibid.
4. Fidler, G: From crafts to competence. Am J Occup Ther 35:567–573, 1981.

2

Occupational Genesis: The Evolution of Human Activities

He who sees things grow from the beginning will have the best view of them.—ARTISTOTLE

Philosophers have long understood that knowledge of the past contributes to an understanding of the present. This chapter describes the genesis of human occupations from earliest times to the modern era. This sequence allows us to understand the meaning of activity for human survival. These ideas are relevant for occupational therapy, because they allow us to see the continuity from traditional to modern activities and highlight the importance of cultural relevance in providing therapeutic activities. Occupational genesis describes the process of change over time that considers the history and development of occupation and their implications for practice.

ACTIVITIES FOR SURVIVAL

From their beginnings, as individuals and as groups, human beings have occupied themselves in activities that have kept them alive. From the earliest times, the activities of humans have contributed to their growth and well-being and assured their survival during and beyond their lifetimes. Early peoples pursued and trapped and dug their food; they found shelter in natural crevices and caves; they nurtured their young. They mastered these tasks through trial and error, adapting them as they went along, passing the necessary skills on from one genera-

tion to the next. As they refined their skills, they ensured the survival of their groups, passing their heritage beyond them into the modern era, where remnants of these activities remain today.

MASTERY

For activities to be fully effective and to benefit the individual or the group, they must be meaningful and they must be performed skillfully. Developing skill in tasks is an ongoing commitment of human beings. People are forever refining their skills in unlimited directions. By sharpening their skills, first in activities called play, then during work and leisure, they continue the process of learning throughout their lives. New skills are learned through play and exploration, by modeling the behaviors of others, and from instruction.[1-3] Regardless of how learning takes place, as time passes, responsibilities demand that skills be sharpened. In the process, mastery is achieved.

Mastery is that level of performance in which automaticity takes over the routine aspects of tasks. When routine tasks can be performed automatically, new and complex extensions of those tasks can be attempted. Mastery describes skilled performance from which higher levels of creative thinking and performance can emerge, because the underlying subskills that enable the performance do not require conscious attention. Automaticity allows skills to develop on ever more complex levels because conscious attention is released to resolve more complex questions of performance. Automaticity is enabled by innate and habitual systems and is at the heart of occupational genesis.[4,5] Human beings strive to become more skilled, that is, more automatic, in the mundane aspects of activity so that their efforts can be directed at further problem solving, further development.

Mastery can be developed in all aspects of performance: riding a bicycle, learning to write, or cutting facets in diamonds. During the development of mastery, both universal and unique skills are learned. Each individual builds on skills common to all, seeking personal direction. In time, special and often unique abilities are gained through a combination of talents and opportunities. As they master increasingly specialized aspects of performance, people assume individualized roles, enabling them to take responsibility for themselves and for others in their families and their societies.

People have engaged in this developmental process from the beginnings of history; they remain engaged in activities meaningful for themselves and their community to this day, although the nature of their tasks and tools has changed over time and will continue to change in the future (Fig. 2–1).

EVOLUTION AND PRODUCTIVITY

Whether people learn to do activities by experimentation or by instruction, whether they are engaged in play, work, or the special effort called leisure, human beings

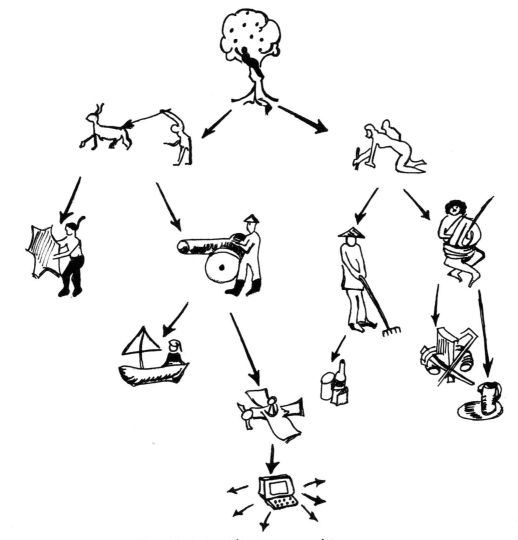

Figure 2–1. Specialization is an evolving process.

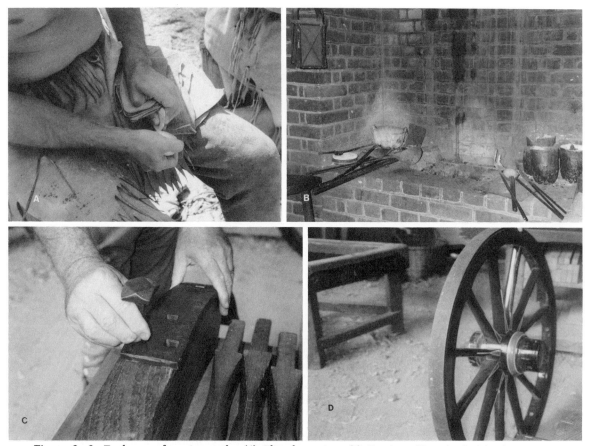

Figure 2–2. Tools-manufacturing tools. (*A*) Flint knapping. (*B*) Forging. (*C* and *D*) Wheelwrighting.

are recognized by their products and their tools. Indeed, even their tools are their products. Not only do human beings create their own tools, but they also create tools to create tools (Fig. 2–2). In the process, humans have increased their productivity by geometric proportions.

Increasing their skill in productive and meaningful activity is part of the purposeful nature of human beings. Ever searching for new solutions to questions of their own design, human creativity and individuality in these pursuits sets us apart from the other inhabitants of this earth. People are continually developing better, more efficient means of doing things, and the objects with which they occupy themselves are an integral part of the purposefulness to which they are dedicated. Human beings' continual engagement in purposeful activity is part of an evolutionary adaptive process in which we have engaged since we first evolved as erect primates several million years ago (Fig. 2–3).[6]

That evolutional process resulted in a remarkably specialized creature. As humans stood erect, they could view their environment more effectively, at the same time freeing their hands for manipulative tasks. Without needing their forelimbs for support, their use of tools increased. With time and experience, their tools became increasingly refined. The opposable thumb with which

humans were gifted enhanced their ability to perform skillfully, as did their unique-handedness and inventive communication. The incredible specialization and dexterity of the human hand both enabled and was enabled by the process of tool use, while the ability of human

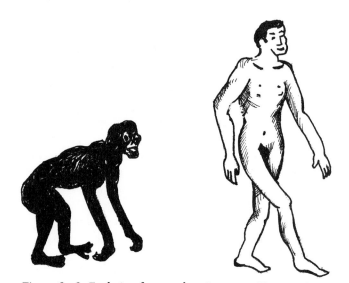

Figure 2–3. Evolution from early primates to *Homo sapiens*.

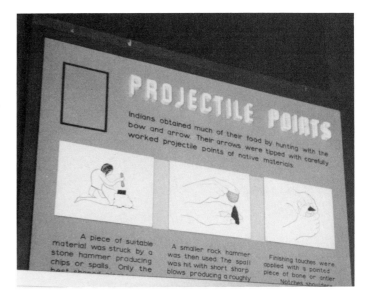

Figure 2–4. Arrowheads used by Northwest American Indians.

beings to speak and develop language allowed them to share ideas. The use of tools contributed to physical changes, whereas changes in structure enabled further adapted tool use.[7] This reciprocal process resulted from and contributed to the efforts people made toward their survival as social beings. Development and evolution mirrored one another in this change process, in the many environments that people encountered and then mastered, and in which they survived.

A GENESIS OF ACTIVITIES

Ancient peoples met their survival needs by searching their world for food, shelter, and understanding. They found their tools and their salvation among the rocks (Fig. 2–4), the clay, the vegetation, and the animals about them. They understood their world through its objects, and what they did not understand, they interpreted according to the things with which they were familiar. Animals were their food and their totems. They looked to them for nurture and for comfort. The spirit world was as real for them as the world that they could see, hear, and feel (Fig. 2–5).

Early humans honed their skills in collecting the bounty of their world, and when that world ceased to yield its produce, when the spirits were no longer kind, they moved on to other lands to hunt and gather anew. The metaphor of Eden represents that process, that ancient trip from the land of plenty to the land of adventure. Human beings came to inhabit mountains, islands, frozen tundras, and rain forests, accommodating to each new environment with inventive approaches. As they expanded their vistas and collected their food supply, they increased their skills in using nature's yield. They build their homes of stone, skins, ice, and wood. They

refined their hunting tools. Rocks and sticks became knives, lances, and many other tools. They wove baskets to carry their possessions. They used the skins of animals to keep themselves warm and dry. They harnessed fire to cook their food and to alter the properties of the clay

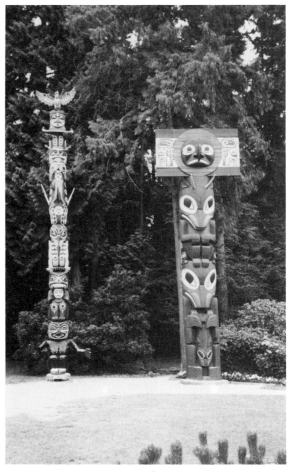

Figure 2–5. Totem poles, Vancouver, BC.

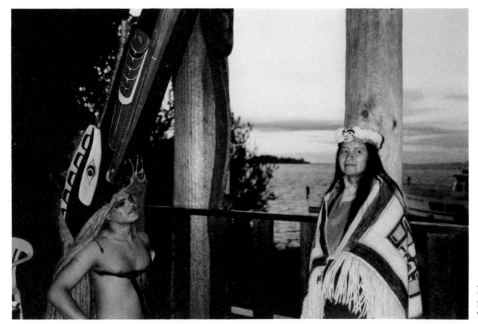

Figure 2–6. Clothing and ceremonial headdress worn by Tlingit tribe, Tillicum Island, Seattle, WA.

they dug. Despite their problems in overcoming the elements and the natural restrictions of their many worlds, they worked out functional methods of transforming the bountiful produce about them into useful products for survival. In ever-evolving new and creative ways, they used the yield of the hunt for food, for clothing, and for shelter (Fig. 2–6).

The land provided everything they needed. No portion was unused. The skin and the bone were as valuable as the flesh. Insects, birds, fish, and four-legged creatures fed and clothed them. Roots, leaves, fruits, and flowers kept them well. People respected their world for its ability to provide for their needs. They developed rules for the use of the earth and its bounties, and honored their gods by respecting their environment. They harvested their world with care, so that it would reciprocate.

Experience taught people what methods were successful in adapting their world to their needs, and equally significant, what methods were futile and dangerous. They learned the differences between toadstools and mushrooms. They knew which berries to eat, and from which to make dye. They knew the season of hardship and how to prepare for it. They taught the successes and failures to their children, who in turn practiced and refined these skills in play until they too could take their place in the responsible life of their community. They developed ceremonies to recognize this transition from childhood to adulthood. In every society they developed customs, rules, laws, and religions, all in an effort to protect themselves from their environments, from one another, and from the unknown.

Whether in the role of hunter or of gatherer, each individual's contribution to the group depended on the ability to care for the self and to care for others, for these two elements are united. Self-care is an individual's basic contribution to society. Once people master the skills of personal survival, others are no longer burdened by their care. By participating in life's activities, ancient peoples honed their skills in caring for themselves and for others, for their lives depended on their mutual survival. Independence was, as it is now, a form of responsibility for self, and in the process, for others. A society that must care for its people beyond their ability to reciprocate is burdened.

Both play and work were devoted to learning and performing mutual caring skills. The role of children was to learn the skills they would need as adults so that they would not become a burden to others in a world of hard-earned resources. They threw sticks, ran, played games, and picked berries, all to hone their skills for the responsibilities they were about to assume. Inland and on sea, in high altitudes and low, in tropical, temperate, and frozen lands, people gained the skills they needed to survive by adapting the raw materials they had at hand to new forms. They made fibers into yarn and then into cloth; they made grasses into cooking implements. Human curiosity and creativity enabled this process. Engaging in this adaptive process, simple but inventive people became increasingly complex, as did the world in which they lived.

Following their early traditions as harvesters of a natural environment, they learned to husband animals so that their need to hunt was lessened and their food supply secured. They moved from place to place to feed their animals and themselves. They made rocks malleable, learning to call them metals and altering them in remarkable ways (Fig. 2–7). They created durable goods and traded them from one community to another. They learned to harness the soil so that it would yield crops, securing themselves to the land. They built homes of stone, wood, and steel. They made machines that could do the work of humans, and they made machines that did things that humans could not do. In time, they broke the barriers of gravity and sound (Fig. 2–8).

These inveterate hunters and gatherers set their sights on new environments, new worlds, always seeking more effective ways to get the job done. However, among the gains made, failures continued. Humans created fouled environments, hazardous waste, and weapons that endanger the hunter to the same extent as the hunted. The rapid changes produced by their remarkable inventiveness did not allow humans to solve the problems they were creating in sufficient time to teach these methods to their children to keep them safe. They lost sight of the knowledge that survival encompasses the total group in mutual concern and caring. It began to appear as if people did not need one another.

Skills and behaviors that function well in one environment are not necessarily successful in another. Habits die hard; even unsuccessful ones. The remarkable skills of human memory and communication are an advantage and a disadvantage at once. Humans tend not to forget. What has once been learned is not easily unlearned.[8] Memory retains the bad with the good, the obsolete with the adaptive.

Time is needed to ascertain what works for society and what does not in order to make the changes that will best meet humanity's needs. Skills that originally enabled people to survive have remained with us past their usefulness representing a constant conflict between the old and the new. The young rebel, seeking change, while the old cling to the known and proven. Cultural diversity both provokes and stimulates us. Old habits, skills, and artifacts appear in conservative elements of any given community; they are symbols of human history. Customs reflect the past. Museums display their evidence. Yet, human creativity never ceases to develop new ideas and implements. The relationship between the old and the new must forever be reorganized.

In this process of change from ancient times to the present, imperative tasks become optional; the skills of the artisans become arts. Artifacts remain in the modern world, changed in the role they serve for society, sometimes without a clear recognition of their connection to the past. The arts of survival became the crafts of triviality and frivolity. Baskets that carried the means of life

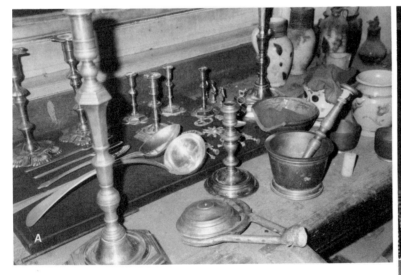
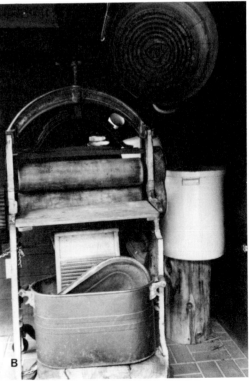

Figure 2–7. (*A*) Candlesticks, spoons, mortar, and pestle (1700s). (*B*) Tub, washboard, and wringer (1800s).

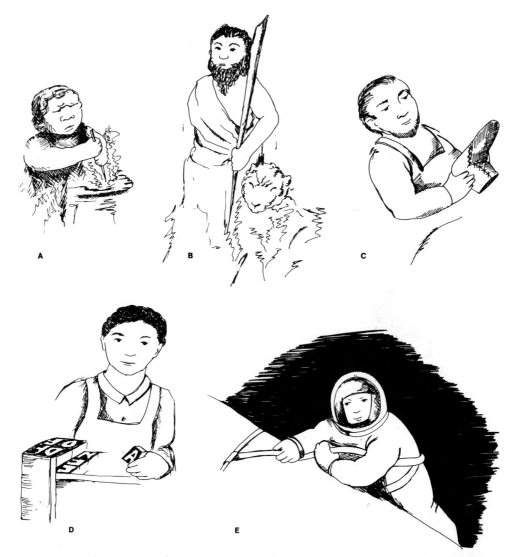

Figure 2–8. The transition of activities used (*A*) by hunters/gatherers, (*B*) by nomads, (*C*) by town dwellers, (*D*) in industry, and (*E*) in the space age.

now adorn the table containing papier maché replicas of the fruits of yesteryear. Survival and artistry are no longer one.

Modern people still work to survive, but their jobs, tools, and materials differ from those of the ancients. Skills continually develop in response to the demands of the modern world. In an age of rapidly advancing obsolescence, the known is adapted creatively into the new. Biodegradable plastics, genetic engineering, and nuclear disarmament portend solutions to what at times seem to be insurmountable problems. Time allows people to address problems of great complexity with new and creative solutions. Discoveries, inventions, and new systems contribute to an ever-changing world of increasing complexity. Old and new overlap, ever conflicting, provoking anxiety, as the world diminishes in size.

Telephone, radio, television, satellites, and spacecraft allow communication with the farthest reaches of the

world and beyond. The community is composed of larger and larger numbers of people, yet their direct relationships diminish. Neighbors are strangers as their dependence on one another becomes more remote. As a result, individuals appear less significant to their group, and when this occurs, their own self-worth is diminished. Unquestionably, as the tribe expands, its connections dilute; it can survive without its members being aware of their interdependence. The global village has strangers in its midst (Fig. 2–9).

PURPOSEFULNESS IN ACTIVITY

Those who work as though they were unconnected to others in their group, or who engage in a kind of fractioned work where they lack control over their own efforts, are not likely to understand the value of their

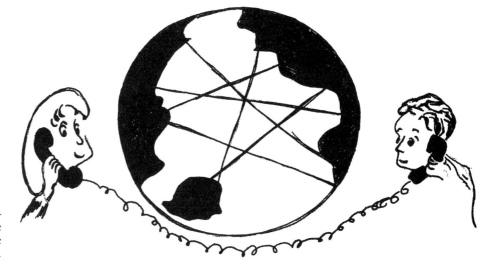

Figure 2–9. The term "global village" is used to describe the ease of communication now possible among peoples all over the world.

skills to the larger society. If their worth is devalued, by themselves or by others, they are limited in their ability to fully contribute to their society. To be a healthful, productive member of society, one must be recognized as contributing on some level. One must feel effective or competent[9,10] in order to remain purposeful and productive.

Purposeful activity depends upon the intent of the laborer.[11,12] If workers' intentions are limited by their lack of connection to their society, then their productivity is compromised as their feelings of purposefulness are reduced. Without a sense of purpose, one's productivity and sense of self are at risk, along with one's health. The views individuals hold about themselves are critical to their health. Because individuals and their societies are inextricably bound up in each other's welfare, health and safety are of a larger dimension than customarily viewed.

These views about the relationship between activity and health and their implications for society were of great concern to the scholars and social activists who founded occupational therapy, as their world experienced the effects of the industrial revolution. Many of these same issues continue to concern the modern world.

Modern society has risks that the ancients could not have imagined. The job of human beings continues to be to resolve these problems, just as they have done in every other point in time. New environments continue to bring new problems that demand new solutions, ever fulfilling the evolutionary promise of human beings. It remains to discover those solutions, just as it will as long as people continue to inhabit the earth.

REFERENCES

1. Reilly, M: Play as Exploratory Learning. Sage, Beverly Hills, CA, 1974.
2. Welker, WI: An analysis of exploratory and play behavior in animals. In Fiske, DW and Maddi, SR (eds): Functions of Varied Experience. Dorsey, Homewood, IL, 1961, pp 175–226.
3. Bandura, A: Psychological Modeling: Conflicting Theories. Aldine-Atherton, Chicago, 1971.
4. Breines, EB: Origins and Adaptations: A Philosophy of Practice. Geri-Rehab, Lebanon, NJ, 1986.
5. Breines, EB: Genesis of occupation: A philosophical model for therapy. Aust Occup Ther J 37:45–49, 1990.
6. Leakey, R and Lewin, R: Origins Reconsidered: In Search of What Makes Us Human. Doubleday & Co, New York, 1992.
7. Washburn, SL: Tools and human evolution. Sci Am 203:63–75, 1960.
8. Koestler, A: Insight and Outlook: An Inquiry into the Common Foundations of Science, Art and Social Ethics. Macmillan, New York, 1949.
9. Fidler, GS: From crafts to competence. Am J Occup Ther 35:567–573, 1981.
10. White, RN: Motivation reconsidered: The concept of competence. In Fiske, DW and Maddi, SR (eds): Functions of Varied Experience. Dorsey, Homewood, IL, 1961, pp 278–325.
11. Breines, EB: An attempt to define purposeful activity. Am J Occup Ther 38:543–544, 1984.
12. Breines, 1986, op. cit.

3

The Doing Philosophy

DEWEY AND LEARNING

Healthy relationships between individuals and their societies are established through their responsibility to one another. Establishing such relationships in the society in which he lived was a concern of John Dewey. This renowned philosopher of pragmatism, educator, and social activist taught at the University of Chicago, where the philosophy of pragmatism was so influential in the early 20th century.

Pragmatism is a phenomenological philosophy that allows no distinction between subjectivity and objectivity. It is grounded in the dialectical or relational concepts of Hegel, the German philosopher, and the evolutional concepts of Darwin. It recognizes the inextricable influences on each other of the mental and physical aspects of human beings, their artifacts, their environments, and the societies and times in which they live. Pragmatism is called a philosophy of evolution, time, and history. It is widely recognized as the only American philosophy and is foundational to sociology, education, psychology, and occupational therapy.[1]

To seek adaptive solutions to the problems of his changing society as it dealt with the industrial revolution, Dewey developed a model for education based on humanity's genesis of occupations. He organized this model along the lines of the foregoing discussion. Dewey structured students' education according to a genetic framework stimulated by "active occupation" and "purposive activity."[2] His plan was to contribute to the learning and citizenship of his students by connecting them to the roles they would play in society. He did this by engaging his students in purposeful interdependent activities.

Dewey believed that children learn best when they recognize their contribution to a larger effort. He facilitated this recognition by involving them in serial tasks that required active effort in purposeful activities of mutual benefit. He believed that if students understood their contribution from a historical perspective, they would recognize their responsibilities to society and, hence, their own importance. That recognition came from active involvement in collaboration with others.

To reverse what he and others in his world saw as the ill effects of the industrial revolution, Dewey designed a teaching method that he hoped would change society in positive directions. He believed that workers who engaged in labor practices such as assembly-line work could not be certain that society recognized the contribution of their labor, because their contribution was not clear, either to themselves, or to others. Working on a portion of a product for which one does not contribute to its design, in which one's own work cannot be distinguished from that of others, or where one can easily be replaced because the level of skill needed to perform is minimized, can limit pride in one's own efforts. Furthermore, this diminished sense of personal importance can impact negatively on one's personal health and, reciprocally, on the health of society.

Dewey attempted to counter these negative influences by using active occupation as a teaching tool. From their earliest school years, children in his Laboratory School learned by doing, by engaging in tasks of a collaborative nature.[3] By engaging in the activities of past societies, students learned that they were contributing individuals, part of a productive group whose contributions were needed and valued, and part of a historical thread relating the past to the future.

In creating this model, Dewey was bound by the principle of "learning by doing." He recognized that it was through active occupation, purposeful activity, and creative, adaptive problem solving that human beings reduced their uncertainty and mastered the skills they needed to develop as individuals and as societies. Learning one's place in this continuum would build children's awareness of the relationship of work to society's progress and welfare. It was his intention that this realization would aid them as adults, when they would be expected to contribute to their own society.

According to Dewey's educational model, the earliest grades engaged in activities that had been survival tasks for early peoples. They began their education by using the same tools and ideas as the hunters and gatherers. By replicating a microcosm of a society, the students were expected to gain the skills and knowledge that earlier peoples had acquired as they solved the problems of their world.

In each subsequent school year, a more complex society was introduced, with new skills to master. Students learned new ideas and skills in virtually the same sequence that societies had developed them. Just as ancient peoples generated new skills and knowledge from ideas that came before, so the children in Dewey's Laboratory School learned, re-creating activities that societies had used to survive. In their natural historical sequence, students learned each craft as it was needed to meet the goals of their microcosmic society, their class. For example, they used simple counting skills to complete the tasks used by hunters and gatherers. Then, in constructing replicas of the kinds of wooden buildings agricultural peoples used, they learned to compute numbers and measure angles. As each skill was learned in turn, concepts built on concepts, just as new ideas and skills had been incorporated into societies' occupational tasks throughout history.

By adapting, by using the tools necessary to perform new tasks, and by cooperating in these tasks, students recapitulated the physical, mental, and social learning that had taken place throughout history. They learned as they worked that from the shelter provided originally by caves, and later by leather and cloth dwellings, humans ultimately developed architecture and its inherent measurement of distances and angles, and they grasped the significance of this knowledge for society through actual experience. By experimenting with tangible items, students learned how ideas developed, evolved, and related to one another in each society in turn.

Dewey expected that as students actively learned this sequence of occupational genesis, they would apply this knowledge to the modern world. They would come to understand that the labor in which they would soon engage as adults was their own means of contributing to society, similar in responsibility to the activities required in ancient times.

DEVELOPMENT, WORK, AND PLAY

Learning comes from the past and leads to the future. Just as societies learn, learning is a lifelong developmental process for the individual, during which creativity and competence alternate in the development of skill. Development is a form of change, a form of adaptation and evolution. G. Stanley Hall, Dewey's teacher, recognized this relationship between the past and the present in his famous principle, "ontogeny recapitulates phylogeny" (Fig. 3–1). According to this principle, changes that take place within any one lifetime mirror the changes that have taken place over the millennia.[4] The one-celled creature that evolved millennia ago is like the fertilized ovum; over time, from each, the adult human evolves or develops. One sequence occurs in terms of centuries; one in terms of months. Each, however, follows the same sequence: a living organism bound in a fluid environment, a creature bound to the earth by gravity, a four-legged creature, and one that stands erect. Past, present, future—the means by which the nature of time is measured—are inherent in these genetic themes.

Time is the thread that passes from the past to the future. From ancient to modern times, this continuous thread can be understood through the changes that take place within each lifetime as individuals develop and learn. This learning process, this sequence, is provoked by the questions that life's experiences offer and by the nature of human beings to explore for answers to those questions. Dewey termed this pursuit of knowledge, humanity's "quest for certainty."[5]

The trek human beings follow in their continual pursuit of knowledge is devoted to the resolution of doubt. For each individual, this journey begins with the earliest activities of childhood. This struggle toward knowledge starts with the tools with which nature has endowed human beings: their physical and mental makeup in all its parameters, their innate capacities for learning and performance. Upon this inherited foundation, learning and development proceed, stimulated by exploration and environment. Childhood is filled with a curiosity satisfied by the continual pursuit of skill and knowledge. From this perspective, work and play are two sides of the same coin. Both are directed at achieving independence and social responsibility from childhood through adulthood (Fig. 3–2).

In this pursuit of knowledge, each individual repeats the sequence of the past. Then, from this universal heritage, each person points his or her questions to unique expertise sought through new experiences. The lifelong search for new solutions to ever-more-intriguing questions is reflected in the genesis of active occupation. Activity is the human endeavor that feeds people's souls and meets their needs.

During this search, certain universal qualities can be

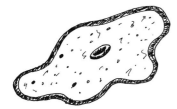

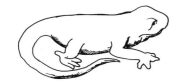

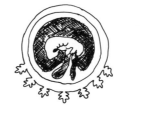

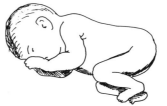

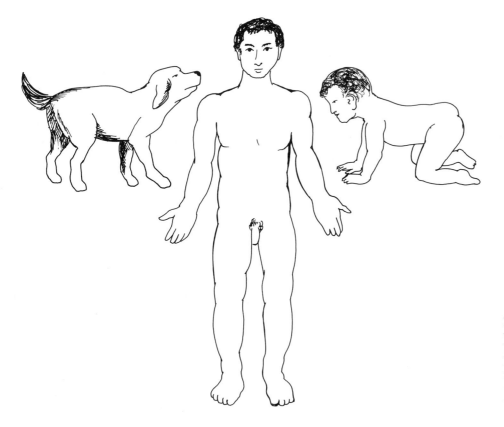

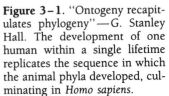

Figure 3–1. "Ontogeny recapitulates phylogeny"—G. Stanley Hall. The development of one human within a single lifetime replicates the sequence in which the animal phyla developed, culminating in *Homo sapiens.*

observed. Each new activity is initially approached with uncertainty. Unfamiliarity with the task and its physical and mental requirements contributes to the uncertainty. In the doing, familiarity and skill develop, mastery is achieved, and in its turn, certainty comes—and with that certainty come feelings of competence, efficacy, and pride. This sequence is the same no matter the task. Questions provoke us to learn. Activities provide the answers. Success in performance results in self-confidence and the willingness to pursue further questions.

When questions are self-induced, as they are when children spontaneously play and explore, the uncertainty of the unknown is countered by the curiosity that initiated the task. Readiness for learning is demonstrated by participation in the search. On the other hand, when uncertainty is imposed by external forces, the resulting anxiety can be defeating. Getting past the anxiety is a growth step, resulting in mastery. Facilitating that growth was the problem Dewey addressed.

According to Dewey, learning should be structured so

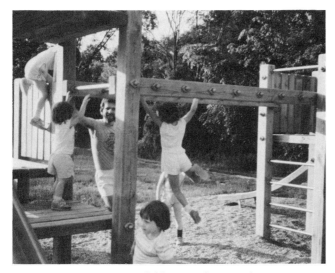

Figure 3-2. Children working at play.

that it can take place in effective and tolerable increments, so that the learner can see the relevance of the problem to his or her life. Readiness, timeliness, and meaningfulness contribute to learning. Learning is best achieved by engaging in activities during which learning can naturally take place, because learning is then more likely to be meaningful and relevant.

When children search for answers at their own pace, many of the tasks they engage in are called play. Actually, many aspects of these activities can also be considered work, in the sense that they are provocative, demanding, and fruitful. Whether called work or play, every task has two elements: (1) an element of ease, skill, and automaticity on which new skills can be established and (2) an element of effort and concentration through which new skills can be acquired. The work of children is to build competencies and to continually acquire new skills in preparation for life's later work. The natural curiosity of children leads this process of growth and development. In this sense, although the work of children is indeed play, their play is also work.

As adulthood approaches, additional elements assume importance. Social responsibility emerges as the driving force for learning. Toys come to be described as tools, games as part of a larger social effort. Work comes to be considered those activities society demands from responsible individuals. All too often, work is viewed as difficult and unpleasant, whereas play is seen as easy and fun. This view is simplistic and false. Both work and play can be fun and difficult, so this differentiation is not only inaccurate, but it also restricts understanding. For example, leisure activities, the play of adults, can be more demanding than any other effort. Workaholics may not be aberrant; they may just be having a good time from the satisfaction their efforts provide.

All activities, whether engaged in by children or adults, retain the same two elements: automatic and deliberate action. Various theorists have used related terms to describe alternate phenomena that parallel deliberate and automatic actions (Table 3-1).[6-9]

Each task requires attention, deliberation, query, and purposefulness, while at the same time, other elements of the same tasks are done habitually, reflexively, automatically, and confidently.[10,11] These two elements, automaticity and purpose, serve action in a fluctuating, reciprocal, dialectical process. Without this communication between the demanding and the comfortable, the new and the familiar, whereby some aspects of performance are purposeful or deliberate and some are reflexive, habitual, or automatic, skill cannot be gained, and development cannot proceed. Without the release of play and the value of work, human beings would be void of growth and satisfaction.

Play and work, the activities of life, represent both a relational and an evolutional scheme in which all people in every society and of all ages have engaged throughout life and throughout lifetimes. Growth and evolution are enabled by this search for skill. Activities people have learned and repeated over the millennia are sometimes work and sometimes play—but always meaningful, or we would not do them.

It is this last rule that must be heeded. Regardless of the task in which one is occupied, be it play or work, it will offer no fruit to the tree of life unless it is meaningful to the person engaged in that activity. It must be part of one's quest for certainty, or it will lack meaning for living, for learning, or for therapy.

THE CHICAGO SCHOOL

Dewey[12] influenced his colleagues in these beliefs in learning by doing, active occupation, and purposive activity. Among his colleagues at the University were George Herbert Mead, pragmatist philosopher and sociologist; Paul Triggs, influential in the American Arts and Crafts movement; Rabbi Emil Gustave Hirsch, phi-

Table 3-1. DELIBERATE AND AUTOMATIC ASPECTS OF BEHAVIOR FLUCTUATE IN ACTIVITY

Deliberate Elements	Automatic Elements
Cortical	Subcortical
Conscious	Unconscious
Cognition	Perception
Purpose	Habit
Will, volition	Reflex

Table 3–2. HISTORY OF THE PHILOSOPHY OF OCCUPATIONAL THERAPY

1880s	*Pragmatists*			
	Chicago		**Massachusetts**	
	Dewey, Mead		James, Peirce	
1900s	*Social Activists*			
	Chicago		**Massachusetts**	
	Dewey		James　(Nat'l Ment. Hyg. Soc.)	
	Addams　(Ill. and Nat'l Mental Hygiene Societies)			
	Lathrop　(Illinois Mental Hygiene Society)			
	Hirsch　(Illinois Mental Hygiene Society)			
	Meyer　(Illinois Mental Hygiene Society)			
1908	*First OT School*			
	Chicago School for Civics and Philanthropy			
	Hirsch } founders			
	Lathrop			
	(Addams' Hull House)			
	Slagle, student			
1917	*Founders of N.SPOT*			
	Chicago	**Baltimore**	**New York**	**Canada**
	Slagle	Dunton	Tracy	Kidner
		(Slagle)	Barton	
			Gladwin	
			Johnson	
		(Meyer)		
		(Hirsch)		

From Breines, E: Origins and adaptation: A philosophy of practice. Geri-Rehab, Inc., Lebanon, NJ, 1986, p 277, with permission.

losopher, theologian, reformer, and, along with Julia Lathrop, founder of the first school of occupational therapy; Lathrop and Jane Addams, both of Hull House fame, prominent in the settlement house movement; Dr. Adolf Meyer, renowned pathologist, psychiatrist, medical educator, philosopher of occupational therapy, and with William James and Eleanor Clarke Slagle, as well as Hirsch, Addams, and Lathrop, active in the mental hygiene movement (Table 3–2). The mental hygiene movement was devoted to applying Dewey, Mead, and James' principles of pragmatism to health, education, and social welfare, and it was the immediate precursor to the founding of occupational therapy as a profession.[13,14]

These scholars and social activists were bound together in the belief that active occupation was beneficial to the health of individuals and society. They advanced Dewey's beliefs in the interdependent relationship of people and their community in areas described today as social work, special education, psychiatry, and occupational therapy.

Dewey's principles were world famous. It was natural that his community would adopt his beliefs and apply them to their individual interests. If students could be educated through the use of "active occupation and pur-posive activity" (Dewey's own language), then these same tools could be used to advance the health of modern society.[15] In effect, this was the goal of the mental hygiene movement, which Addams, Hirsch, Lathrop, Meyer, and Slagle promoted with vigor in the form of occupational therapy.

EVOLUTION AND ADAPTATION

Primary practices, to which occupational therapy still subscribes, stem directly from the theory of evolution, Dewey's foundational premise. Grading of activities and adaptation based on activity analysis are the original and essentially unique principles and practices of occupational therapy. They are based on the assumption that change results in response to environmental influences, and that change can be elicited by using these same factors. Therapists skilled in adapting activities and environments continue to use these concepts to heighten performance and improve health.

The evolutional premise assumes that in nature, serendipity, or unplanned events, fosters change. Environmental conditions can foster or restrict the growth of organisms. When the organism responds positively to environmental influences, it adapts, survives, and progenerates, whereas maladaptive organisms expire and become extinct. This phenomenon is called evolution, and it results in what Darwin called "survival of the fittest."[16] These effects of environment can also be observed relative to societies. Early peoples used their environments creatively. When they could adapt as needed, they survived. Many did not.

These ideas about evolution did not entirely meet with acceptance. The idea of translating a concept drawn from biologic theories to social applications was heavily criticized. These criticisms should be examined from today's perspective, because some of them can be understood in ways that had to be unclear to these early scholars, given the level of scientific understanding at the time. Evolution is not a simplistic concept, and it cannot simply be dismissed. Newer theories reveal what theorists and critics of the past might not have recognized.[17]

Darwin's idea of survival of the fittest can be understood today according to newer scientific theories about genetics that were not known when the theory of evolution was proposed.[18,19] We now recognize that changes in organisms and their environments do not directly lead to the inheritance of adaptive traits, as Meyer's understanding of eugenics led him to believe. Eugenics, an idea prevalent early in this century, held with the belief that an individual's experiences were directly inheritable. Adolf Meyer's concern that his mother's melancholia was inheritable stems from his belief in eugenics.

However, environments and behaviors do not simply cause living things to evolve. Although adaptation can be stimulated within an individual, for a trait to be inherited, a capacity for change must be genetically available. Interestingly, nature has endowed species with the wherewithal to recruit unused capabilities in adaptive ways to assure their continued survival. In other words, species retain broader genetic capabilities than are evident within one individual, or even one generation. These capabilities are recruited when environmental conditions enable them to be adaptive.

Piaget[20] describes several of these natural phenomena in *Behavior and Evolution*. Existing species can withstand unfavorable conditions by producing some offspring with the qualities necessary to survive in one environment and some that could survive under different circumstances. For example, moths indigenous to London existed as black creatures in a city of soot-covered buildings; they emerged as white when the buildings were cleaned. Individual moths did not change from black to white. Neither did they change genetically because of the environmental change. The genetic makeup of this creature allowed offspring of each sort to be produced in all generations, but the survival of each variety depended on the specific environment. Black moths survive in a black environment and white ones survive in a white world because their predators are unable to find them in an environment that inhibits their detection (Fig. 3–3). A previously maladaptive variety of this species of moth can now survive under new environmental conditions. Consequently, the species, not a specific organism, survives and evolves by adaptation.

Whether the pragmatists understood this complex process is not the issue here. Rather, evolution served as a metaphor for understanding survival and the related issue of health. They essentially proposed that education serves the same purposes for society as does genetics for a species. Learning can be inherited, not in the biologic sense, but in the social sense. It is passed on from generation to generation. Education serves adaptation, the adaptive organism exhibits health, and with health the group survives. For the pragmatists, biology and sociology were totally united. This was their premise: Individuals and society are totally and inseparably bound in each other's welfare. Education, health, individual, and society are necessarily one.

Darwin's view of evolution was prevalent at the turn of the century. When the theory of evolution was proposed, it was a generative force in the development of world knowledge. It structured the thinking of the pragmatists, educators, and social activists who appreciated the relevance of this theory for social growth and learning. They were intrigued by the evolutional, historical, and developmental process by which societies endowed their offspring with knowledge and skill, enabling them to adapt to unpredictable environments and circumstances. Ulti-

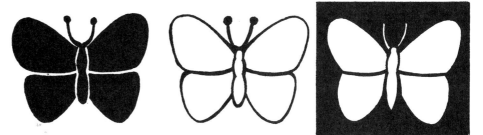

Figure 3–3. Black moths and white moths are distinguishable from their background when the background is contrasting but indistinguishable when their color matches their environment. This adaptive characteristic serves as a protective mechanism for their survival.

mately, as a direct descendant of the concept of evolution, adaptation became the premise on which occupational therapy practice was built.

PRINCIPLES OF PRACTICE

The early proponents of occupational therapy adopted the principle of evolution and adapted it to the promotion of health and learning. Disabled individuals could be enabled through adaptation, and, through the acquisition of health, could become contributing members of society. Adaptive performance in individual and social benefit was understood to be relevant for children and adults, regardless of deficit. This model of social evolution was applied to health in a unique and creative form, established as occupational therapy.

By modifying tasks or the environment in tolerable increments, diminished capabilities can be recruited to enhance function. By making objects heavier or lighter, simpler or more complex, by changing their texture, or by positioning them to increase or reduce physical demand, functional performance can be altered, ability can be enhanced, and disability remediated or circumvented. Therapists demonstrated that skillful manipulation of the human and nonhuman environment can influence performance and contribute to learning and health.

From the beginning, therapists were instructed in these adaptive skills. Being able to structure an experience so that it is enticing, intriguing, and not fear-provoking is a special skill that occupational therapists develop. Proficiency in this skill marks the master clinician.

Before arguments about philosophy and theory development falsely questioned the field's status as a profession, occupational therapists were skilled in certain basic techniques.[21] These techniques are founded in evolution and pragmatism, a theory and a philosophy widely recognized as major contributions to world knowledge (Table 3–3). In developing their body of knowledge, therapists did not recognize the intellectual advantage these integrated themes provided, but they developed them nevertheless. Even though these foundational concepts were not explicitly identified by the profession's founders, occupational therapy adapted these philosophic, theoretic, and tangible tools to the service of humanity.

Table 3–3. PHILOSOPHY, THEORY, AND PRACTICE ARE RELATED

Philosophy	Theory	Practice
Pragmatism	Evolution and adaptation	Occupational therapy

Because of their encompassing education and training in the functional and dysfunctional realms of mind and body and their awareness of tools, materials, and tasks, occupational therapists remain the only professionals equipped to comprehensively perform activity analysis, grading, and adaptation. Foundational skills in analysis and adaptation are used to improve functional performance in persons with disabilities. Individuals with problems can be enabled to rise above their limitations, contribute to their own independence, and assume responsibility for themselves and others to the highest level of which they are capable. *Enabling function* became the essential theme of practice.

REFERENCES

1. Breines, EB: Origins and Adaptations: A Philosophy of Practice. Geri-Rehab, Lebanon, NJ, 1986.
2. Dewey, J: Democracy and Education: An Introduction to the Philosophy of Education. Collier-Macmillan, Toronto, 1916.
3. Mayhew, KC and Edwards, AC: The Dewey School: The Lab School of the University of Chicago, 1896–1903. Appleton-Century, New York, 1936.
4. Koestler, A: Insight and Outlook: An Inquiry into the Common Foundations of Science, Art and Social Ethics. Macmillan, New York, 1949.
5. Dewey, J: The Quest for Certainty: A Study of the Relation of Knowledge and Action. Minton, Balch, New York, 1929.
6. Freud, S: General Psychological Theory. Collier, New York, 1963.
7. Ayres, AJ: Sensory Integration and Learning Theory. Western Psychological Services, Los Angeles, 1972.
8. Meyer, A: The Collected Papers of Adolf Meyer. Winters, EE (ed). Johns Hopkins Press, Baltimore, 1952.
9. Slagle, EC: Training aides for mental patients. Arch Occup Ther 1:11–17, 1922.
10. Breines, 1986, op. cit.
11. Penrose, R: The Emperor's New Mind: Concerning Computers, Minds and the Laws of Physics. Oxford, New York, 1989.
12. Dewey, 1916, op. cit.
13. Breines, 1986, op. cit.
14. Cohen, S: The mental hygiene movement; the development of personality and the school: The medicalization of American education. Hist Educ Q 23:123–149, 1983.
15. Dewey, J, 1916, op. cit.
16. Darwin, CR: The Origin of Species by Means of Natural Selection. Macmillan-Collier, New York, 1859.
17. Leakey, R and Lewin, R: Origins Reconsidered: In Search of What Makes Us Human. Doubleday & Co, New York, 1992.
18. Keller, E: A Feeling for the Organism: The Life and Work of Barbara McClintock. WH Freeman, New York, 1983.
19. Piaget, J: Behavior and Evolution. D. Nicholson-Smith (trans). Pantheon, New York, 1978.
20. Ibid.
21. Fidler, GS: Professional or nonprofessional. In Occupational Therapy 2001. American Occupational Therapy Association, Rockville, MD, 1979.

4

Therapeutic Activities: Yesterday and Today

A HISTORICAL PERSPECTIVE

Throughout history, active occupation has been associated with healthfulness. Purposeful activity, work and play in all its forms, is recognized as both body building and mind healing.[1-3] This long-standing belief in the therapeutic qualities of activity was adopted by the earliest occupational therapists, even among those who did not necessarily agree with the pragmatists' perspective. During the same period that the Chicago network developed, the physicians Herbert Hall, William R. Dunton, Jr., and others, demonstrated the value of activity for promoting health. Yet, the pragmatists' beliefs in adaptation prevailed in the first schools of occupational therapy, possibly because Dewey's principles were of great interest to educators.

Educating nurses, social workers, teachers, and artisans about the healthful properties of activity, and teaching them the methods and skills associated with this belief, would prove to have far-reaching effects. Susan Tracy in Boston and Rabbi Emil Hirsch and Julia Lathrop in Chicago began their schools. Each were conceptually allied with Dewey. Tracy's beliefs were made clear in her explicit quotation of Dewey's principles: "By occupation I mean a mode of activity on the part of the child which produces or runs parallel to some form of work carried on in the social life."[4] Occupation was established as the contribution the individual made to society, and this contribution was viewed as healthful to both.

Hirsch and Lathrop's Chicago School for Civics and Philanthropy, the first school in which active occupations as therapy were taught, held its classes at Hull House, where Dewey and Lathrop taught philosophy each week and where Slagle studied and later taught. It is no surprise then that Dewey's Laboratory School activities found their way into Hull House, and vice versa, and into occupational therapy education as well. Weaving, basketry, leatherwork, and claywork, the principle constructional occupations of ancient peoples, became part of the early occupational therapy curriculum, along with the more industrialized activities of metalcrafts, carpentry, and printing. The genesis of occupations was established in these early schools as a tool for health.

Remnants of these skilled activities, these crafts, remained evident in practice and education, despite the fact that their existence created a dilemma for some as time passed. The rationale for the use of crafts was not entirely clear, and their use was hard to defend in the scientific arena of practice.

Influences of the medical community shifted the focus from crafts to a measured scientific approach, as if science alone could assure health. Practice became streamlined. Sanding boards no longer held sandpaper, and there was no wood to sand. Clay was converted to Theraplast. The use of leather lacing diminished. Standardization increased. Purposeless exercise increased, and productivity diminished. Task groups became talk groups. Basket weaving became a dirty word. The pride in purposeful activity in which the profession was grounded was more difficult to find and to defend, while at the same time defense became necessary. The character of practice changed.

Despite these changes, curricula retained crafts as therapeutic tools, while the profession's underpinning in Dewey's philosophy of social evolution remained largely unnoticed. The communal memory of therapists, along with their certainty about the value of crafts as therapeutic tools, assured their survival in the schools, despite the absence of an explicit rationale to guide their selection.

The influences of the Arts and Crafts and moral treatment movements,[5-9] along with the pressures of the medical community, clouded the perspectives of educational and social pragmatism and occupational genesis that Dewey and his colleagues offered.

When craft activities were survival tools, the skills they required were mundane daily tasks, of no particular note. Their products were unremarkable, other than that they enabled life. As with most ordinary yet important things, the objects of daily living are rarely viewed as remarkable, even when they are endowed with considerable artistry. Things people do on a daily basis usually are considered mundane and without special merit. However, focusing on and mastering the mundane became the occupational therapist's unique and remarkable skill.

Unfortunately, skill in dealing with the ordinary was largely unrecognized and unrewarded, just as ordinary things ordinarily are. Consequently, as time passed, views about practice changed. Too often, the activities of social evolution became the arts and crafts of trivial pursuit. With new materials and new ideas, baskets were no longer considered vital implements. They became ornaments devoid of the purposes for which they originally had been designed, and their meaningfulness diminished.

Two divergent thrusts for therapeutic activity were established while the identical media were retained. One was devoted to artistry, expression, diversion, and leisure. The other was committed to improving function. When crafts were emphasized for their role as art forms instead of their role in tasks of daily living, objects once vital to survival became tools of diversion. This emphasis on diversion was undervalued and eventually was largely passed off to other therapeutic communities. Meanwhile, leatherwork, basketry, weaving, and woodcrafts were used to strengthen. Neither purpose fostered any understanding of the contribution of these modalities to society's welfare in their original form, as Dewey and his colleagues had intended. The notion of self-care diminished to the narrow perspective of bedroom and bath. The tools of practice were no longer viewed in their entirety as part of a global concept.

Without an encompassing, overarching principle, therapists were confused as to their professional identity. This dilemma became compounded as time passed. The inventiveness that thrust humanity into the technologic age caused uncertainty for therapists and society at large, for they were unprepared for such changes.

When occupational therapy was developed early in the 20th century, it was a time of industrial and social revolution, with the disruption ordinarily associated with marked change. In an effort to return to the character of earlier times when people understood the meaning of activities for their very survival, crafts were promoted as therapeutic tools. The return to handcrafts in an industrialized era was an attempt to heal society. Despite society's expressed wish to return to "the good old days," it could not revert to its earlier forms, any more than time could be turned back. The world continued to advance, with all of its emerging changes. Inventions came faster and faster, solving some social problems and introducing others. Industry improved the availability of goods, while at the same time it brought new health and social problems. The new developments became part of everyone's lives. Change became an expectation, obsolescence a rule. Values and interests continued to change in ways that could not have been anticipated by the social reformers and founders of occupational therapy.

In keeping with society, the profession was torn by divisive forces. Crafts, the traditional tool of occupational therapy, were suspected by some and defended by others. Attempts were made to explain the profession's devotion to this familiar tool. At the same time, new tools began to replace those that could not be validated, either philosophically, scientifically, or consensually. The differences between the old tools and the new were met by reaction, argument, and defensiveness.[10-14] Questions about identity and professionalism emerged, while the meaning of purposeful activity was discussed, defined, and repeatedly redefined. The essential theme of occupational therapy was masked by uncertainty, expressed in part as a search for a philosophy.[15]

As modern society altered its tools, skills, and values, so did practice, further enhancing the profession's dilemma. Without a clear understanding of the rationale for the use of activities as originally conceived by Dewey and his Chicago colleagues, crafts were kept in the curriculum while their use in the clinic diminished, creating a broader rift. Still more incongruent, for many years individualized treatment was emphasized, even when numbers of patients were together. A focus on therapeutic groups reemerged in the 1960s but not in the societal context offered by Dewey. In the absence of an encompassing rationale, this additional difference furthered the identity crisis. Practice in different areas of specialization began to look markedly different from one area to another, contributing to the questions of identity voiced in the profession.

As people's lives changed, so did the health arena. Changes in society's tools and tasks were reflected in the clinics. New equipment and responsibilities emerged, because in order to return people to the modern world as functional individuals, they needed to live among modern implements. Occupational therapists rose to the oc-

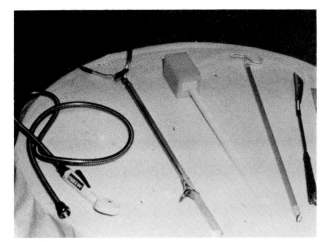

Figure 4–1. Adaptive equipment.

casion. They took the newest inventions and adapted them to therapeutic purposes. They adapted keyboards and telephone holders. They devised one-handed insulin dispensers and used Velcro in creative ways (Fig. 4–1). They entered patients' homes and developed methods of using household gadgetry to enable independence. They jumped into the technologic era without hesitation. They installed computers and became skilled in their use, adapting them to create new opportunities for patients whose needs never could be met before. Therapeutic equipment, systems, and procedures emerged from the technologic revolution as a natural consequence. From switch-operated toys to augmentative communication, using adaptive formboards and environmental control systems, therapists graded activities and adapted environments, enabling patients in ways that could not have been foreseen.

Despite their difficulty in articulating their beliefs, their early principles of adaptation and occupational genesis served therapists well, even as their tools changed. Therapists began to recognize that the inventions of human beings that offer them purpose are the profession's tools of therapy, whether the tools stem from the past or lead to the future, as long as they bring meaning and purpose to people's lives. Occupational therapists applied their traditional skills to activities that are meaningful to their patients in the modern world.

THERAPEUTIC PRACTICES

Throughout the history of the profession, despite the changes in society and its tools, certain of occupational therapy's fundamental practices remain unchanged. These practices are called activity analysis, adaptation, and grading of activities.

Activity Analysis

Human beings engage in widely different activities. The variety of these activities reflects human uniqueness, which is all the more evident when one has sustained a trauma or birth defect, encountered disease, or when the inevitable decline associated with aging limits function. Each individual has capabilities and limitations that exist in unique combination and impact on performance. Still, people engage in all types of activity.

Activity has been described as healthful or therapeutic. Activities have been used to remediate deficiencies, but in order to use activity as a therapeutic tool, its thorough analysis is mandatory. Activity analysis is the process of determining the multidimensional elements involved in performing any task. Activities encompass minute aspects of tasks to comprehensive occupations. They range from areas of personal care to industry. Activity analysis is used to identify all the dimensions of any given task, regardless of the type of activity. Analysis of the complex effects of activity on the body and mind determines how activity can be used as therapy.

Some aspects of activity are tangible; others are subjective. All are interactional. People and things impact on one another in activity. Activities demand a combination of interrelated elements. For example, to write a paper requires physical and mental ability, writing implements, and the ability to communicate with the audience. To perform skillfully requires a refined interaction between mind and body, time and space, and the contributions of others. Activity analysis permits each element to be considered alone as well as in relation to each other element, and to the whole.

Activities use all aspects of the sensory and motor systems, stimulating these systems in unlimited variety and combination.[16,17] Vision, hearing, touch, taste, smell, and the proprioceptive and vestibular systems interact, contributing to a refined awareness of environment. Beyond these major sensory systems, each sense is composed of subsystems that further refine how the world is known. For example, the multiple subsystems of vision determine size, distance, color, movement, speed, dimensionality, and relationships. Touch informs the individual about temperature, texture, pressure, structure, size, and density. Each sense is endowed with specialized cells that contribute information. The integration of these elements allows one to make sense of the world.

In addition to sensory stimulation, there are perceptual, cognitive, and emotional effects inherent in activity. For example, sweet smells are pleasant, whereas pungent smells are noxious. Each can trigger memories of past events or bias perspectives of current and future experience.

Activity analysis considers the implications of activity on memory and motivation, along with its effects on muscles and joints. For example, the resistive activity of bread kneading, while strengthening muscles, can elicit memories of past kitchens and warm caring. Each sensory element contributes to performance, while the influence of each varies according to its role in performance. Activity analysis exposes these differences and sets the groundwork for the use of activity as therapy. Essentially, activity analysis determines the extensive and particular effects of any given activity on mind and body, as they relate to the tangible world, and to other people in that world.

Consequently, activity analysis is a complex and extensive process that examines all the effects that activities can potentially provide, simultaneously and sequentially. Therefore, it corresponds to a systems model in which feedback is an essential element,[18] a model grounded in pragmatic philosophy.

Since activity effectively connects each and every dimension of performance, a relational phenomenon exists. No aspect of the relationship can be viewed entirely in isolation. Simultaneously, individuals interrelate with objects and environment, as well as with other people. For example, to cook a meal requires physical and mental ability, ingredients and utensils, and a family to come to dinner on time. With any feature missing, this activity is unsuccessful. To clarify this vastly complex phenomenon, a special language is needed.

Those elements related to the mind and body of the individual are *egocentric*. Those elements external to the individual having to do with space and time and tangible objects (otherwise known as the "nonhuman environment" and temporal dimension) are *exocentric*. Those elements having to do with relationships or communication with others are *consensual*.

Activities that involve objects generate egocentric and exocentric relationships. Activities that involve communication with others establish egocentric and consensual relationships. Meaningful activities integrate these three elements in a relationship described here as "wholesome," for their holistic character (Fig. 4–2).

Wholesomeness is also a way of describing health. Many views of health have been described,[19] but only this relational phenomenon reflects the pragmatists' perspective: purposeful, active occupation stimulates the interaction of the mind and the body with the tangible, temporal, and social environments toward adaptive or functional ends. This model was advanced by the mental hygienists Adolf Meyer, Eleanor Clark Slagle, Jane Addams, Julia Lathrop, Rabbi Emil G. Hirsch, and William James. "Holism," in the sense described here, is the underlying premise for the use of activity as a tool to enhance or structure health. It is from this philosophy that the therapeutic use of adaptation and grading of activities derives (Table 4–1).

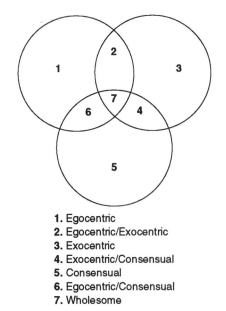

1. Egocentric
2. Egocentric/Exocentric
3. Exocentric
4. Exocentric/Consensual
5. Consensual
6. Egocentric/Consensual
7. Wholesome

Figure 4–2. Relationships elicited through activity.

Adaptation and Grading of Activities

Adaptation is the tool therapists use to enable function. Occupational therapists adapt the environment, tools, the medium, and positioning. Egocentric adaptation can be in the form of strengthening, positioning, learning, or other factors that affect the mind or body. Exocentric adaptation uses adaptive equipment, modified environments, altered speed, and graded activities, all influences of time and space. Consensual adaptation can be through the use of such activities as structured task groups, parent training, or vocational preparation. Adaptation of each or all of these areas can induce change in performance.

Since egocentric, exocentric, and consensual elements all interact in performance, any and all can be adapted in

TABLE 4–1. ANALYSIS OF "MAKING A GAME"

Activity	Classification
1. I thought about making a game and reached over to get the materials.	Egocentric
2. I started to manipulate the materials.	Egocentric/exocentric
3. The materials on the table were of many textures and colors.	Exocentric
4. The lab assistants put the materials on the table.	Exocentric/consensual
5. A team designed and constructed the game.	Consensual
6. Each member of the team cooperated to make the game.	Egocentric/consensual
7. We had fun!	Wholesome

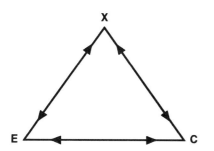

Figure 4–3. Egocentric (E), exocentric (X), and consensual (C) elements influence one another. The relationships among these elements are represented by the lines. Occupational therapy changes these relationships by influencing (adapting) any or all of these elements: mind/body, time/space, or social interactions.

unrestricted combinations. Change in any of these elements influences the others (Fig. 4–3). For example, by adapting the environment, the patient with physical disorders can be enabled to dress, work, and pay taxes. By changing physical and mental abilities and spatial, temporal, and social environments, the individual can be taught to act in new ways. Adaptation of any of these can enhance functional performance.

Grading of activity is a form of adaptation. Grading enhances performance by adapting activities in selected increments. All activities can be graded to heighten performance. For example, to build muscle power, one might gradually increase the resistance necessary to perform a given task by adding weights, the time spent at the activity, or the number of end products to be completed. To heighten concentration, one might eliminate distractions or control and introduce them in tolerable limits. Grading can be offered in positive or negative directions. One can introduce fewer or more interventions, smaller or larger demands, and so on. The type or extent of grading is determined by professional judgment. Grading activity can enhance the healthy functioning of mind and body by building skill in areas of functional performance. The purpose of grading activity is to increase the capacity of individuals to perform in tolerable increments in order to bring them to their highest level of performance for their age or other descriptor.

Use of activity analysis, adaptation, and grading was and remains the foundation for practice. Applying these principles to purposeful activity became the skill of the occupational therapist.

REFERENCES

1. Hopkins, H and Smith, H (eds): Willard and Spackman's Occupational Therapy, 8th ed. JB Lippincott, Philadelphia, 1993.
2. Meyer, A: The Collected Papers of Adolf Meyer. EE Winters (ed). Johns Hopkins Press, Baltimore, 1952.
3. Peloquin, SM: Occupational therapy service: Individual and collective understandings of the founders, Part 1. Am J Occup Ther 45:352–363, 1991.
4. Tracy, SE: Studies in Invalid Occupations: A Manual for Nurses and Attendants. Whitcomb and Barrows, Boston, 1918.
5. Bing, RK: William Rush Dunton, Jr., American psychiatrist: A study in self. EdD dissertation, University of Maryland, 1961.
6. Bing, RK: Eleanor Clarke Slagle lectureship: Occupational therapy revisited: A paraphrastic journey. Am J Occup Ther 35:499–518, 1981.
7. Levine, R: The influence of the Arts-and-Crafts movement on the professional status of occupational therapy. Am J Occup Ther 41:248–254, 1987.
8. Peloquin, 1991, op. cit.
9. Peloquin, SM: Occupational therapy service: Individual and collective understandings of the founders, Part 2. Am J Occup Ther 45:733:744, 1991.
10. Breines, EB: An attempt to define purposeful activity. Am J Occup Ther 38:543–544, 1984.
11. English, C., et al: On the role of occupational therapists in physical disabilities. Am J Occup Ther 36:199–202, 1982.
12. Fidler, GS: From crafts to competence. Am J Occup Ther 35:567–573, 1981.
13. Huss, AJ: From kinesiology to adaptation. Am J Occup Ther 35:574, 1981.
14. Trombly, CA: Include exercise in "purposeful activity." Am J Occup Ther 36:467–468, 1982.
15. American Occupational Therapy Association: Resolution 531. AOTA, Rockville, MD, April 1979.
16. Breines, EB: Perception: Its Development and Recapitulation. Geri-Rehab, Lebanon, NJ, 1981.
17. Gibson, JJ: The Senses Considered as Perceptual Systems. Houghton Mifflin, Boston, 1966.
18. von Bertalannfy, L: General Systems Theory. George Braziller, New York, 1962.
19. Smith, J: The Idea of Health: Implications for the Nursing Professional. Columbia University Press, New York, 1983.

5

An Occupational Genesis Model for Activity Analysis

All activity is multifaceted, and each activity demands a different set of capabilities. For example, sawing wood is a resistive activity, requiring motivation, focused vision, unilateral strength, range of motion, and grasp. Tossing a large ball back and forth requires cooperation, bilateral coordination, ambient vision, and spatial orientation. Recognizing these characteristics is a fundamental skill for occupational therapists.

To use activities therapeutically, therapists must master activity analysis. Activity analysis allows therapists to examine a life task so that each element of the task can be adapted to improve function. Analyzing the components inherent in activities is the most basic tool of practice, allowing therapists to draw on them for evaluation and treatment. Activity analysis underlies the development of standardized and phenomenologic assessment tools (Table 5–1), and enables therapists to identify the performance elements in every activity and to isolate and combine them so that they can offer appropriate therapeutic experiences. Learning to analyze activity is the skill that ushers the student into the realm of therapist. Once this skill is learned, it marks the special way an occupational therapist thinks about the world.

Occupational therapists improve patients' functional performance by designing activities in such a way as to place adaptive demands on performance. Because patient's problems and interests vary widely, therapists must have a working acquaintance with a great many activities from which they can draw. In the clinic, these activities are analyzed along with the assessment of pa-tients' functional abilities, to determine which tasks will enhance function in the dysfunctional individual. Because of the wide variability in patients' capacity to perform, the assessment of dysfunction is beyond the scope of this book. Here, the focus is on activity and its analysis, whether self-care, play, work, or leisure, for these are universal occupational performances, regardless of age or ability.

Educators in the past have designed various ways to teach this skill. Some have made activity analysis a fragmented technical endeavor. To avoid this fragmentation, the occupational genesis model is consistent with the egocentric, exocentric, and consensual concepts described in Chapter 4. The egocentric element concerns physical and mental capacities. The exocentric element includes objects and environment in space and time. The consensual element addresses the implications of social interactions. Each of these elements is evident in all activity. All activities require physical and mental abilities in combination with the tangible components of that activity, along with the influences of others. All activities demand interactions among these egocentric, exocentric, and consensual elements. Each of these elements interact, regardless of whether the activity is entitled work or play. Relationships exist between egocentric and exocentric elements; egocentric and consensual elements; exocentric and consensual elements; and among egocentric, exocentric, and consensual elements (see Fig. 4–3). Activity analysis examines isolated aspects of these elements as well as their interactions.

Table 5-1. STANDARDIZED AND PHENOMENOLOGIC ACTIVITY-BASED EVALUATION TOOLS

Tool	Activity
Standardized Evaluation Tools	
Allen Cognitive Levels (ACL)	Ceramic, leather, wood
Bay Area Functional Performance Evaluation (BAFPE)	Drawing
Goodenough House Tree Person	Drawing
Scorable Self-Care Evaluation	Computer
Phenomenologic Evaluation Tools	
Azima Battery	Drawing, ceramic
BH Battery	Drawing, mosaic
Build-a-city, Build-a-farm	Paper
Carolyn Owens Activity Battery	Paper
Clark Clay Test	Ceramic
Comprehensive Assessment Process	Mosaic, paper
Comprehensive Evaluation of Basic Living Skills	Cooking
Diagnostic Test Battery	Drawing, leather, ceramic, wood
Fidler Activity Laboratory	Drawing, paper
Elizur Test of Psych-Organicity	Drawing
Gillette Battery	Ceramic, mosaic
Goodman Battery	Drawing, ceramic, mosaic
Gross Activity Battery	Drawing, ceramic
Interest Check List	Cooking, drawing, leather, ceramic, mosaic, needlecraft, wood
Jacobs Prevocational Skills Test	Cooking, leather, wood
Kinetic Family Drawing	Drawing
Lafayette Clinic Battery	Paper
Magazine Picture Collage	Paper
Mattis Dementia Rating Scale	Drawing
Milwaukee Evaluation of Daily Living Skills	Needlecraft
O'Kane Diagnostic Battery	Drawing, ceramic
Perkins Title Task	Mosaic
Shoemyen Diagnostic Battery	Ceramic, paper
Street Survival Skills Questionnaire	Cooking
Tiled Trivet Assessment	Mosaic
Work Adjustment Program	Drawing, wood

RELATIONSHIPS AMONG ELEMENTS

Egocentric and Exocentric

Egocentric elements are those of the mind and body. Exocentric elements are those related to objects and the environment. The relationship between egocentric and exocentric elements includes readiness to perform, exploration of environment, and manipulation of objects.

Readiness to perform follows a developmental sequence in which foundational skills emerge. These skills include:

1. Head turning
2. Tracking
3. Righting
4. Rolling
5. Creeping
6. Crawling
7. Sitting
8. Grasping
9. Standing
10. Walking
11. Climbing
12. Running
13. Speech
14. Jumping
15. Hopping
16. Skipping

These foundational skills are innate and acquired, are achieved in a largely predictable developmental order, and are the underpinning for performance.

Prior to engaging in activity, one must exhibit readiness to perform. That is, one must have matured enough both neurologically and physically to engage in an activity. Readiness to perform governs the interaction between the individual and objects. For children, this interaction is manifested in play. Play enables and is enabled by the development of foundational skills and is therefore vitally connected to readiness to perform

Table 5-2. TOYS AND READINESS

Children's Toys	Readiness Levels (see list on page 29)
Mobiles	1–2
Blocks	1–8
Beads	1–8
Tops	1–8
Crayons	1–8
Pull toys	1–10
Balls	1–12
Puzzles	1–13
Tricycles	1–15
Jump rope	1–16

(Table 5–2). Foundational skills are preliminary to engagement in all human endeavors and are acquired as development takes place. They enable the exploration of environment and manipulation of objects.

The relationship between egocentric and exocentric elements, that is, exploration and manipulation of the environment, is seen in the use of tools. Because the tools of children primarily are toys, play with toys develops skills children will need in order to manipulate and operate tools as adults (see Table 5–2).

Adults build on skills gained in childhood and use tools more typically associated with grownup activities. Adult tools can include:

1. Devices used for the manipulation of objects and materials, such as
   A. Cooking implements
   B. Hammers
   C. Needles
   D. Pliers
   E. Electric saws
2. Devices used for recording time, space, and events, such as
   A. Measurement instruments
   B. Calculators
3. Devices used for communications, such as
   A. Writing implements
   B. Telephones
   C. Computers

Egocentric and Consensual

The *relationship between egocentric and consensual elements* is manifested in interaction and communication, rule development, and role development. Communication is evident in all human interactions: pairs, small groups, large groups, and societies. Members of groups openly and tacitly agree to perform in certain acceptable ways. Groups develop open and unspoken rules to clarify and govern communications among their members.

They decide what roles are to be played within their social groups and who will play those roles. Roles exemplify and determine communications among people.

Children begin to learn to interact with others from the time they are born, developing many of these skills through play. Adult roles grow from those of children, but become more specialized with maturity, education, and experience (Table 5–3). Egocentric and consensual elements in children are integrated through game playing. Through games, children develop these essential human skills of communication, preparing them for adult roles.

Some games are diadic and some are played in groups. Games follow a developmental sequence as they are learned through play. Their complexity increases with maturity. For example, games include peek-a-boo, clap hands, ring-a-rosie, hide and seek, hopscotch, board games, team games, and organized sports. Beyond game playing, people engage in many other activities that broaden their interactive skills.

Exocentric and Consensual

Exocentric and consensual relationships are inherent in the objects used in every society. Tools, artifacts, residences, and so on, are recognizably cultural. It is incumbent on the therapist to be sensitive to objects and environments congruent with cultural norms to foster wellness.

Wholesome Activities

As people develop, they mature in body and mind, gain skill in the manipulation of objects in their environments, and integrate these elements in life roles. Ordinarily, their activities are age-appropriate. Tasks of childhood and adulthood are characteristically different. However, regardless of age, each activity requires the

Table 5–3. ROLES OF CHILDREN AND ADULTS

Child	Adult
Child	Child
Sibling	Sibling
Partner	Partner
Friend	Friend
Student	Student
Classmate	Classmate
	Parent or grandparent
	Worker
	Team or member
	Spouse or other
	Educator
	Representative

integration of the individual, the environment, and others in a feedback loop. That is, activities require interactions with objects as well as people. Cooking a meal for a family requires mental and physical skills; food and utensils; and sensitivity to the likes, dislikes, and needs of others.

The nature of adult activity tends to change with maturity. Many adults come to find more satisfaction in work-related tasks than in game playing. Some view work as an extension of play. Others view work as a hardship. Work is characterized as a more responsible level of performance, because successful engagement in work provides resources for worker, family, and society. Therefore, activities can be understood to be wholesome in two senses. First, they combine egocentric, exocentric and consensual elements. Second, they can contribute to health.

As skills develop from childhood through adulthood in the pursuit of wholesomeness, new activities replicate the same sequence. Mental and physical skills are brought to bear, first on the tangible environment and then on the social environment, ultimately incorporating them in a wholly relational or interactive system. This can be seen when one learns a new skill such as typing. First the fingers must practice and the mind must remember the locations of the keys on the typewriter. It is only then that skill can meet the needs of a job role.

Essentially, the relationship among egocentric, exocentric, and consensual elements allows occupational genesis to proceed, enabling growth for the individual and for society. Therefore, occupational genesis can be understood in an ontogenetic (developmental) as well as a phylogenetic (evolutionary) sense.

MASTERY

Each new activity is first approached with hesitation, attention, and some apprehension. As skill is achieved, the activity comes to be performed somewhat automatically, with pride of accomplishment. Automaticity can aid or hinder function. When aspects of performance are reflexive or habitual and are adaptive, automaticity is all to the good. For example, when one becomes skilled at writing, it serves as a tool for further knowledge development.

On the other hand, if some aspect of performance is maladaptive, automaticity may need to be modified. Performance can be brought to conscious attention, reverting to a level of automaticity or adaptive disregard, after correction of the maladaptive behavior. For example, if one has acquired a habit such as smoking cigarettes, one may need to review the patterns of that habit to reorganize them before one can change the behavior. Once the behavior has changed, then the new behavior becomes

automatic, contributing to health. These ideas were fundamental to the principles of habit training espoused by Eleanor Clarke Slagle.[1]

Adaptive automaticity is a sign of mastery and is necessary to attain higher levels of function. Mastery is the goal for all tasks and is the key to occupational genesis, for without mastery, learning and development cannot proceed. Until one can type without looking for the letters, one cannot compose without distraction. When performing activity analysis, one should consider whether a given element of performance is automatic or deliberate.

Mastery of Activity Analysis

Skill in activity analysis, like all skill building, is developed with experience. The long list of performance elements may cause the beginner to assume that one needs to recall it in its entirety. On the contrary, such a detailed approach can interfere with the learning that should be taking place. When learning activity analysis, the interactive aspects of activity should be emphasized. The list is meant as an analytical taxonomy, a resource, and a guide. At the beginning, however, learning activity analysis requires attention to detail. The student needs to recognize the elements potentially inherent in each activity being analyzed within a framework for organizing those elements.

Skill at activity analysis must be acquired from experience at doing tasks. Consequently, learning to do many activities is vital to mastering activity analysis. The student should learn to do the activity and analyze it later.

As with all skills, when mastery is acquired, automaticity is achieved. The competent therapist learns activity analysis to the extent that it becomes an automatic skill performed spontaneously in everyday and professional life. This level of skill enables one to choose from an ever-expanding repertoire of tasks—as life demands them and as time and invention bring them within the scope of human endeavor.

THE ANALYSIS

This activity analysis follows the model described earlier in which three elements: egocentricity, exocentricity, and consensuality, are present in all activity. These three elements interact in performance, but for the purpose of analysis and clarity they are analyzed separately.

Each element is listed in Figure 5–1 and includes items commonly addressed in many different forms of activity analysis. That is, the items are not unique; the organization is. Many of the items listed appear in many published and unpublished sources, because forms of activity analysis have been generated by therapists and educators since the profession was established. Where the use of any term may differ from customary use, a definition is provided. Some items are not customarily considered in activity analysis, but because they are aspects of activity of some sort, they have been included to be comprehensive. Activity analysis should be an extensive task so that the potential effects of any activity can be recognized. A blank activity analysis form is provided in Appendix D. This form can be photocopied as needed. Figure 5–1 shows what the form looks like when completed as well as demonstrating how the task of sawing a piece of wood can be analyzed.

This analysis differs from others in that it is consistent with the underlying philosophic foundations with which this book is concerned. This consistent organization should aid students and therapists and make it clear that our foundational philosophy is alive and well in our most fundamental tool of practice, activity analysis.

SUMMARY

Each of the items listed in the analysis has been isolated and defined for purposes of organization and clarity and to fulfill the inherent role of activity analysis, which is intensive examination. It must be remembered, however, that these divisions are artificial; these elements are inseparable in activity itself.

As skill in activity analysis is acquired, it becomes evident that one activity can be used to elicit many different capabilities, and that many activities can be used to elicit the same one capacity. This recognition explains why occupational therapy is antithetical to a ''cookbook'' approach to therapeutic activity. It is hoped that this model for activity analysis will make it clear that occupational therapy's focus on the mundane activities of living require great sophistication beyond the ordinary.

REFERENCES

1. Slagle, EC: Training aides for mental patients. Arc Occup Ther 1:11–17, 1922.
2. Gruber, H and Voneche, JJ: The Essential Piaget. Basic Books, New York, 1982.
3. Freud, S: General Psychological Theory. Collier, New York, 1963.
4. Maslow, A: Psychology of Science: A Reconnaissance. Regnary Gateway, Washington, DC, 1966.
5. Erikson, E: Childhood and Society. WW Norton, New York, 1986.
6. Gilligan, C: In a Different Voice: Psychology Theory and Women's Development. Harvard University Press, Cambridge, MA, 1982.

ACTIVITY ANALYSIS

Activity: *Sawing a piece of wood with a motorized (scroll) saw*

Student: *Norman Askinazi*

Date: *Spring 1993*

EGOCENTRIC ELEMENTS

(all aspects of mind and body)

MIND

Numerous theorists, Piaget, Freud, Maslow, Erikson, and Gilligan among them, have described ways in which the mind develops. These include the development of learning, emotion, and social awareness. The following are various aspects of the mind.

PERCEPTION

Self-Image (identity):

Cutting a shape in a piece of wood with a scroll saw is a complicated activity and when successfully done can enhance one's self-image and contribute to a positive identity.

Body Image:

The coordination needed to cut a piece of wood also contributes to one's body image.

Discrimination:

of self from other person(s):

Wood cutting is usually a solitary activity, yet the ability to cut a piece of wood with a scroll saw may be perceived as a unique ability not shared by other individuals.

of self from other object(s):

Discrimination of one's hands or fingers from the piece of wood is important so that you don't cut your fingers.

Figure 5-1. Sample of a completed activity analysis form. © 1994 FA Davis Company. Breines: Occupational Therapy Activities from Clay to Computers: Theory and Practice.

of body parts from each other (gnosis):

Necessary to unconsciously coordinate movements of shoulder, arm, forearm, wrists and fingers in turning and positioning the wood as you are cutting it.

of objects from one another (stereognosis):

Necessary to feed and turn the wood by using your sense of touch as you visually line up your pencil line to the saw blade.

Figure-Ground:

Being able to differentiate between the figure, the desired piece of wood and the background (the waste piece) means that you can approach cutting from various points as long as you don't cut into and damage the desired piece.

Form Constancy:

Is important as you may constantly turn the wood and it may be oriented upside down or sideways as you are cutting it.

Spatial Orientation (e.g., vertical, horizontal, diagonal):

Necessary to provide orientation as you turn the wood beneath the saw blade.

Laterality (sidedness of self):

Perception of sidedness is helpful in properly positioning oneself to cut wood accurately and safely.

Directionality (way finding):

Once you determine the direction of sawing, it must be followed accordingly.

Memory (recognition):

Relied on to manipulate the wood.

Symbolism:

One may perceive this activity to be symbolic of one's identity if one is a carpenter.

COGNITION (deliberate, focused attention)

Problem Solving:

Is necessary if the blade begins to deviate from the pencil line.

Doubt (wonder):

Curiosity about the likelihood of success in the final outcome of the wood project may provide motivation to continue.

Inquiry:

One may question what level of quality to achieve and match that to acceptable standards of workmanship.

Intellect:

Should have average intellect or better to plan the project and be aware of the dangers of the saw.

Learning:

May take place through cutting out the same shape of wood repeatedly.

Memory (recall):

Remembering safety factors such as keeping fingers away from the blade and holding wood down firmly will prevent unnecessary accidents.

MOTIVATION

Internal Direction (innate drives, e.g., hunger eliciting eating):

Using a scroll saw to be creative in producing a wood project.

Volition/Will (learned intention, e.g., eating as a plan to avoid hunger):

Sawing wood is a completely deliberate activity under conscious control of the individual.

AFFECT/EMOTION

Happiness:

May be arrived at when finishing a cut without any mistakes.

Sadness:

Is possible when one realizes one has made a mistake and ruined the project.

Figure 5–1. *Continued.* © 1994 FA Davis Company. Breines: Occupational Therapy Activities from Clay to Computers: Theory and Practice.

Anger:

Might occur as a response to failure.

DYNAMIC STATES

Alertness:

Is necessary for safety and accuracy in cutting.

Frustration Tolerance:

There is a high potential in this activity for frustration, for example, if the person tries to cut with a dull saw blade.

Self-Control:

Is always necessary around power equipment.

Reality Testing:

Sawing wood is a concrete activity that forces the individual to focus on the physical reality of the wood and the saw.

Gratification:

Immediate:

Staying on the pencil line when cutting.

Delayed:

Cutting a piece of wood is one step in the process of fabricating a completed project.

TEMPORALITY (subjective)

Immediate:

Takes place in the here and now (present).

Distant:

Has both a past and future component.

Figure 5–1. *Continued.* © 1994 FA Davis Company. Breines: Occupational Therapy Activities from Clay to Computers: Theory and Practice.

Speed:

Relative to using a hand saw, a scroll saw is much faster. The cutting itself can be done with speed, planning may take more time.

Sequence:

All preparatory steps and the activity itself follow a logical sequence in time.

Present:

Takes place in the here and now.

Past:

Obtaining the wood and scroll saw precedes cutting the wood.

Future:

Planning ahead and drawing lines is done in anticipation of future cutting.

SPIRITUALITY

Religion:

This activity does not involve religion.

Ethics/Morality:

This activity is well within the standard norms of society. Wood is a renewable source that can be obtained from tree farms.

BODY

Many aspects of the body are essential to activity. Some of these are evident at birth, some are developed according to a predetermined schedule, some are acquired by experience and practice. These components all interact.

PHYSIOLOGICAL

Cardiovascular:

Low to moderate levels of effort are necessary when using a scroll saw.

Figure 5–1. *Continued.* © 1994 FA Davis Company. Breines: Occupational Therapy Activities from Clay to Computers: Theory and Practice.

Respiratory:

Normal breathing levels. Sawdust is harmful to the respiratory system. Wear a dust mask.

Toxicity:

Sawdust is harmful to respiratory system. Wear a dust mask.

Immunological:

No effect.

Allergic:

Some individuals are allergic to sawdust.

Skin Integrity:

Lengthy exposure to sawdust will dry the skin, and splinters are a hazard.

Biorhythms:

The individual may not want to use power tools at low points in circadian cycles.

MOTOR COMPONENTS

Reflexes and Reactions:

Stretch:

Involves muscle spindles that maintain muscle tautness and the desired position of a limb. This unconscious and automatic proprioceptive activity takes place as one is changing the position of body parts in space (mostly in the upper extremity and thumb, but legs and trunk, too) when the individual is turning and manipulating the wood.

Blink:

If the individual is not wearing eye protection and a piece of sawdust gets in an eye, this reflex will be initiated.

Sneeze:

Sawdust may cause sneezing and coughing.

Figure 5–1. *Continued.* © 1994 FA Davis Company. Breines: Occupational Therapy Activities from Clay to Computers: Theory and Practice.

Balance:

Maintaining your center of gravity is required as you stand and shift your weight from side to side; for example, while rotating and flexing/extending the trunk and neck; adducting/abducting the arms; pronating; flexing/extending the elbows; radial/ulnar deviating the wrists when manipulating the wood.

Equilibrium Reactions:

Required when shifting head position by laterally bending and flexing/extending the neck to get a closer look at the wood.

Nystagmus:

Not elicited.

Orgasm:

Not elicited.

Posture and Position:

Prone:

Not ordinarily required.

Supine:

Not required.

Side-Lying:

Not required.

Quadruped:

Not required.

Sitting:

Possible.

Standing:

Customary.

Figure 5–1. *Continued.* © 1994 FA Davis Company. Breines: Occupational Therapy Activities from Clay to Computers: Theory and Practice.

DEVELOPMENTAL READINESS:

All items below are necessary precursors to movement patterns in adults and the activities in which they engage.

Head Turning:

Helpful when cutting wood.

Tracking:

Must be able to follow the position of the wood and blade as wood is being manipulated.

Righting Reactions:

Needed for posture control.

Rolling:

Not applicable.

Creeping:

Not applicable.

Crawling:

Not applicable.

Sitting:

Saw can be operated in this posture, and standing is needed to operate the saw under ordinary circumstances.

Grasp:

Provides readiness in manipulative hand skills used in positioning wood.

Standing:

Necessary.

Walking:

Necessary to approach the saw.

Figure 5–1. *Continued.* © 1994 FA Davis Company. Breines: Occupational Therapy Activities from Clay to Computers: Theory and Practice.

Climbing:

Not applicable.

Running:

Not applicable.

Speaking:

Necessary to interact with others in discussing the availability of the saw or relaying of instructions.

Jumping:

Not applicable.

Hopping:

Not applicable.

Skipping:

Not applicable.

RANGE OF MOTION

Head/Neck:

Flexion of neck while cutting.

Trunk:

Gross and fine movements of the neck, trunk; rotation and slight lateral bending of trunk.

Limbs:

Upper Extremities:

Flexion/extension, abd/add, medial rotation of the shoulder; elbow flexion; pronation; radial and ulnar deviation of the wrist and manual dexterity.

Lower Extremities:

Extension of hips, knees; ankles at 90 degrees.

MUSCLE POWER

Head/Neck:

Fair.

Figure 5–1. *Continued.* © 1994 FA Davis Company. Breines: Occupational Therapy Activities from Clay to Computers: Theory and Practice.

ACTIVITY ANALYSIS

Trunk:

Fair.

_____

Limbs:

    Upper Extremities:

    Good.

_____

    Lower Extremities:

    Good.

_____

Endurance:

Sufficient to stand and work for 15 minutes.

_____

COORDINATION:

Head/Neck:

Needed.

_____

Trunk:

Required between neck, shoulder, trunk muscles, and extremities.

_____

Limbs:

    Upper Extremities:

_____

        Unilateral:

        No.

_____

        Bilateral:

        Yes.

_____

        Symmetrical:

        No.

_____

        Asymmetrical:

        Yes.

_____

    Lower Extremities:

Figure 5–1. *Continued.* © 1994 FA Davis Company. Breines: Occupational Therapy Activities from Clay to Computers: Theory and Practice.

Unilateral:

No.

___

Bilateral:

Yes.

___

Symmetrical:

Ordinarily.

___

Asymmetrical:

Occasionally.

___

Upper and Lower Extremities:

Symmetrical:

No.

___

Asymmetrical:

Yes.

___

Grasp:

Common grasp patterns do not apply. Palmar pressure is used to control wood.

___

Cylindrical:

Not applicable.

mom

Lt. Hand

___

Spherical:

Not applicable.

___

Hook:

Not applicable.

___

Lateral Pinch:

Not applicable.

___

3-Jaw Chuck:

Not applicable.

___

Figure 5–1. *Continued.* © 1994 FA Davis Company. Breines: Occupational Therapy Activities from Clay to Computers: Theory and Practice.

Fingertip Pinch:

Not applicable.

Hand/Arm:

Feeding a piece of wood into a saw blade requires bilateral pronation of the forearms and palms.

Fingers:

Fingers are extended holding the wood flat while thumb and index finger interchangeably (bilaterally) guide the wood into the blade.

SENSORY COMPONENTS

Near Sensors:

Taste (e.g., sweet, sour, bitter, salty):

Not required.

Touch:

Light Touch:

Meissner's corpuscles aid the person in feeling the wood as it is moved.

Deep Touch:

Pacinian corpuscles help when firmly guiding the wood into the blade.

Temperature:

Not a factor.

Pain:

Rarely a factor unless the person gets a splinter, comes into contact with the blade, or loses control of the wood and is struck by it.

Vibration:

The saw and the wood vibrate. The Pacinian corpuscles detect this movement and guide the individual to hold the wood firmly. Auditory and visual input inform also.

Figure 5–1. *Continued.* © 1994 FA Davis Company. Breines: Occupational Therapy Activities from Clay to Computers: Theory and Practice.

Proprioception (movement of body parts):

Upper extremities, trunk, and lower extremities used when cutting.

Vestibular

Movement of Head:

The organs of equilibrium are located in the vestibule and semicircular canals of the inner ear. Sensory input about head movement provides information used to maintain stability and balance when the head is tilted to focus on accurate cutting.

Movement through Space:

Not elicited.

Kinesthesia (integration of proprioceptive and vestibular inputs):

Needed throughout. Adjustments to the position of body parts are important during movement to maintain balance, muscle control, and coordination.

Distance Sensors:

Smell:

Scent Recognition:

Recognizable scent of wood.

Directionality:

Not evident in room full of saws in operation. Is ordinarily obvious when only one saw is operating.

Vision:

Monocular:

Severe liability.

Binocular:

Needed for depth perception, which affords safety in cutting.

Figure 5–1. *Continued.* © 1994 FA Davis Company. Breines: Occupational Therapy Activities from Clay to Computers: Theory and Practice.

Color:

Color of the wood may be a factor in how easy it is to distinguish the blade from the wood.

Contrast:

The contrasting color of the cut line is useful.

Distance:

Near (accommodation):

Needed to envision wood, pencil line, saw blade, work surface, body parts.

Far:

Needed to orient self in room.

Foveal:

Required for precise cutting.

Peripheral:

Serves to alert one to potential hazards in the periphery.

Ambient:

Not required.

Static:

Not useful.

Moving:

Object:

Must follow movement of wood.

Self:

Must recognize movements of hands.

Hearing:

Monaural:

See below.

Figure 5–1. *Continued.* © 1994 FA Davis Company. Breines: Occupational Therapy Activities from Clay to Computers: Theory and Practice.

Dichodic:

Either one or two ears will inform you that the saw is on, the wood is vibrating, or the blade has broken.

Volume:

Noise levels are high, especially if many scroll saws are working at the same time. Ear protection is recommended.

Discriminant (auditory figure ground):

It may be difficult to recognize that one has left the saw on if many scroll saws are operating at once.

EXOCENTRIC ELEMENTS

(all aspects of external space/time and tangible objects, also known as the nonhuman environment and temporal dimension)

OBJECTS (manipulable)

Food:

Not applicable.

Toys:

Not applicable.

Tools:

A scroll saw is needed.

Materials:

Wood is needed.

Equipment:

Scroll saw, extra saw blades, a pencil, and a power outlet are needed.

Figure 5–1. *Continued.* © 1994 FA Davis Company. Breines: Occupational Therapy Activities from Clay to Computers: Theory and Practice.

Furniture:

A solid counter surface.

SPATIAL ENVIRONMENT (ordinarily beyond the limits of manipulation)

Space:

4' x 4' area.

Terrain:

Flat floor, counter, and work surface.

Weather:

Not a factor.

Time Zone:

Not a factor.

TEMPORAL ENVIRONMENT

Past:

Experience makes for efficiency.

Present:

Cutting slowly can slow the process but increase accuracy.

Future:

Installing a new saw blade in anticipation of working more efficiently. There will be a lamp upon completion.

Speed:

Should be regulated for maximum efficiency.

Duration:

Cutting 4 pieces of wood can be done in up to 10 minutes, depending on experience.

Delays:

May occur if a blade breaks.

Figure 5-1. *Continued.* © 1994 FA Davis Company. Breines: Occupational Therapy Activities from Clay to Computers: Theory and Practice.

Rhythm:

Not applicable.

> ## CONSENSUAL ELEMENTS
>
> **(all aspects of relationships or communication with**
>
> **others)**

DYADIC RELATIONSHIPS

Parent/Child:

A parent may cut out a piece of wood for a child to use in a project of his or her own. Using a motorized saw is too dangerous for a young child.

Spousal:

A spouse may request a door stop to be made.

Friendships:

One may lend a friend help with a project.

Employer/Employee:

A contractor may ask a carpenter to cut a piece of wood as a sample for a customer.

Coworker:

May have to share equipment.

SMALL GROUP RELATIONSHIPS

Family:

May panel a room in the family's home.

Friends:

May need assistance with home repair.

Peers:

May offer one a job after recognizing skill.

Figure 5–1. *Continued.* © 1994 FA Davis Company. Breines: Occupational Therapy Activities from Clay to Computers: Theory and Practice.

Coworkers:

Trade tips and inside knowledge gained from experience.

Teams:

Joining in a group effort to build a home.

SOCIAL INTERACTIONS

Communication:

Is necessary in giving and getting instructions.

Cooperation:

Necessary when waiting to use the scroll saw.

Competition:

May occur if certain individuals desire to outdo each other.

Negotiation:

May be necessary to prevent a Mexican standoff, as when people may decide to split the available time.

Assertiveness:

May be necessary when someone jumps ahead of one's turn on the scroll saw.

Compromise:

May occur when there is high demand to use the saw and the suggestion is agreed to cut out only one piece of wood so the next person can have a turn.

SOCIAL RESPONSIBILITY

Caring:

For Self:

When someone claims the right to use the scroll saw.

For Others:

May occur when a person sees that another needs help and offers the use of the scroll saw.

Figure 5–1. *Continued.* © 1994 FA Davis Company. Breines: Occupational Therapy Activities from Clay to Computers: Theory and Practice.

Play:

Not applicable.

School:

Learning the correct way to cut wood with a motorized saw in school can be a valuable addition to one's knowledge and skills.

Work:

The ability to cut wood with a scroll saw may provide society with a necessary service that the individual can get paid to do.

SOCIETAL INFLUENCES

Ethnicity:

Pertinent to cultures that are industrialized.

Customs:

Certain cultures may prefer to shape wood with fire and remain isolated from the industrial world. Gender and class customs may prevail.

Rules:

Conformity in observing social norms applies to all behavior, even wood cutting. Following rules for safety is critical.

Gender Roles:

Cutting wood with a motorized saw is often perceived as a masculine skill and activity although there should be no basis for this.

Peer Pressure:

May be applied when standards of workmanship establish criteria for success in cutting wood.

Economics:

May be a factor if one cannot afford to buy hardwood or an expensive tool like a scroll saw.

Education:

A grade school level of education is adequate to learn to cut wood with a scroll saw.

Figure 5–1. *Continued.* © 1994 FA Davis Company. Breines: Occupational Therapy Activities from Clay to Computers: Theory and Practice.

ACTIVITY TECHNIQUES: STEP-BY-STEP GUIDELINES

6

Folkcraft

Handcrafts were survival tools for ancient peoples.
Handcrafts offer modern leisure skills.
Handcrafts are used as therapeutic tools.

Folkcrafts originated to fulfill the self-care needs of ancient peoples. As skills developed, these tools of survival were refined into art forms (Fig. 6–1), and art and craft were united with function.

Regardless of their different regional experiences, human beings developed remarkably similar skills. Pots, baskets, fabrics, and other artifacts are found in all cultures. In fact, these artifacts define a culture. Creative and adaptive variations of these crafts arose in different environments around the world. Natural flora, fauna, and terrain, differing from place to place, structured the ideas of these early artisans and can be seen in the designs many different cultures imprinted on their works.

When function merged with beauty, craftsmanship and artistry became indistinguishable. Today, many of these crafts remain with us, although their purposes have largely changed. We no longer depend on these crafts for our daily needs. Crafts have become arts and leisure activities, and judging by the current public interest in hobbies, craft guilds, and craft fairs, many of these activities are still meaningful to people today (Figs 6–2 and 6–3). These tasks from the past have many uses in today's world. Some are functional, such as the dinnerware with which we eat; others are exclusively ornamental, like beaded necklaces. Society places a value on the well-crafted project, although perhaps for different reasons than in the past.

This section describes a selection of folkcrafts, showing how activities in which the earliest people engaged remain relevant both for modern life and for therapy (Fig. 6–4). The crafts described here are simple examples from many places around the world and are suitable for the beginning learner, whether student, therapist, or patient.

Learning these activities will introduce the beginner to unfamiliar materials, tools, and techniques. This will give students the opportunity to develop skills in activities that have traditionally been used as therapeutic tools. It is hoped that students will come to recognize the relationship between these crafts and the activities of daily living of early peoples. Once it is understood that making crafts used to be considered self-care activities, then the estrangement between crafts and the modern activities of daily living should vanish.

Aside from the therapeutic implications, exposure to these creative activities should whet students' appetites for the pleasures that come with developing expertise in these crafts. Perhaps one or more of these activities will enchant you, just as they did our ancestors, leading you to develop sufficient skill to fill your own leisure hours with satisfying endeavors.

> Whatever their derivation, all handcrafts demand problem solving, physical ability, orientation, and perceptual constancy. They offer feedback from the tangible environment, as well as personal and social feedback from the evident successes of a completed work. For these reasons, crafts have been used as clinical tools since the profession of occupational therapy was established.
>
> Learning how to do activities is prerequisite to using them therapeutically. To become a skilled practitioner, one needs to learn many activities, because they are the tools of therapy. Learning the activities described here can provide the beginning therapist with a repertoire of skills on which to build as experience is gathered.

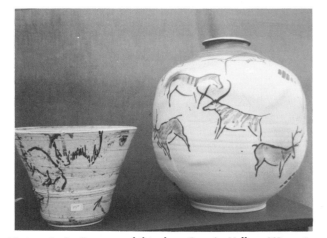

Figure 6–1. Pottery exhibited at Peter's Valley, NJ, artist unknown.

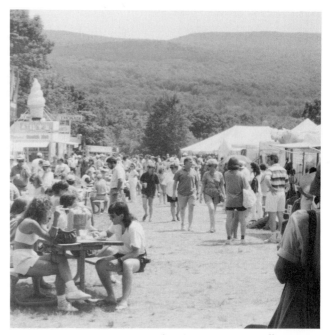

Figure 6–3. Visitors to crafts show at Peters Valley, NJ.

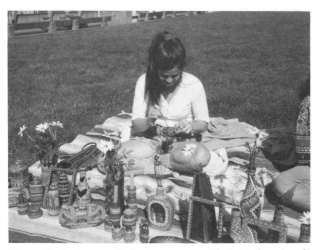

Figure 6–2. Artisan displaying wares at Pike's Market, Seattle, WA.

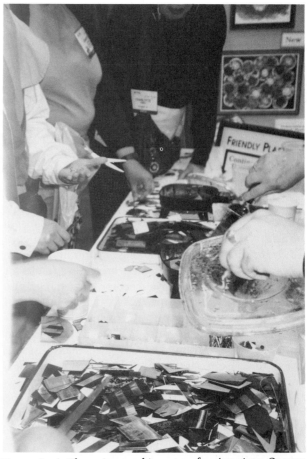

Figure 6–4. Therapists working at crafts, American Occupational Therapy Association Conference, Seattle, WA.

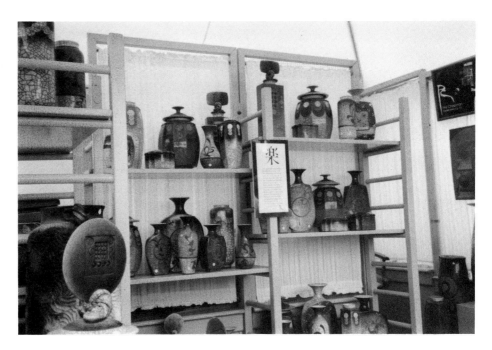

Figure 6-5. Pottery exhibited at Peter's Valley, NJ, artist unknown.

CLAYWORK OR CERAMICS

Times and Events

Clay is a plastic, malleable material dug from the earth. A technology that developed from earliest times allowed this unstructured medium to be transformed into receptacles for cooking, carrying, and many other purposes. Because of their durable nature, ancient examples of these items have been found throughout the world. These artifacts delight archeologists, anthropologists, and others because they reveal the character of the people and cultures from which they came.

Pottery, china, and porcelain, all made from clay, are used today for dinnerware and other household items. The production of ceramic ware, whether for purposeful or decorative uses, has become an art form (Fig. 6-5). Refinement of the basic ceramic process has been improved by modern chemists, engineers, and manufacturers for many industrial purposes, illustrating how old materials come to be used in new ways.

> Working clay requires dexterity and strength, making it useful for improving hand function. At the same time, this unstructured medium offers an opportunity for imagination, creativity, and expression (Fig. 6-6). It is used widely as a projective technique and assessment tool in mental health clinics. Its appeal to children makes it an ideal medium for expressive play.

> Clay is a messy craft, which makes the activity fun for some and distasteful for others. When working with clay, wear appropriate clothing so that the experience can be enjoyed without reservation.
>
> Clay dries out the skin, so hand cream is suggested after washing up. Be aware of skin lesions and allergies, and follow appropriate precautions. Rubber gloves can be used if necessary, but most people enjoy touching clay with their bare hands.

Special Terminology

Wedging. A procedure for eliminating air from clay.
Bats. Plaster of paris rounds on which clay is worked.
Pot. Generic term for receptacles made of clay.
Slip. Liquid clay; used for pouring into molds.
Mold. Plaster of paris form into which slip is poured to produce identical shapes.
Fire(ing). The process of heating clay at high temperatures to make it durable.
Kiln. High-temperature oven for firing pots.
Cones. Ceramic objects that melt at predetermined temperatures so that kiln temperatures can be monitored by observing which cones collapse.
Stilts. Objects used to stack pots in the kiln so that they do not touch other surfaces during firing.
Greenware. A clay pot, dried, before firing.
Bisqueware. A pot after firing; unglazed, porous.

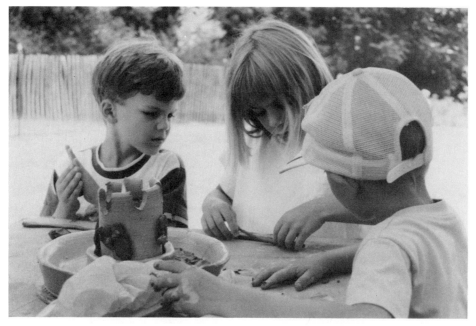

Figure 6–6. Children using clay in expressive play.

Glaze. A finish applied to greenware or bisque for coloring or other surface alteration. When applied to bisque, glaze renders it nonporous. Transparent glazes alter the surface composition without altering color.

Potter's wheel. Revolving equipment, either foot or electricity driven, that permits potters to manipulate clay with their hands.

Drying rack. Clay should be thoroughly dry before firing. Drying should be slow to avoid cracking. Pieces should be covered with a damp cloth to retard drying and placed on a rack.

Wedging Clay

You will need:

Clay
Wedging board or oil cloth

Air pockets in clay pots can cause the pots to explode when they are fired. Not only is the piece being constructed at risk, but other pieces fired at the same time are also vulnerable. Therefore, air should be removed from clay before using it. This is done by wedging the clay.

1. Construct a wedging board of plaster and wood; stretch a wire tautly across it (Fig. 6–7).
2. Form a ball of clay about the size of a softball.
3. Push the clay down onto the wire, cutting the ball in half.

4. Throw one half on top of the other onto the plaster, with the cut edges perpendicular to the surface.
5. Lift the clay; cut it in the opposite direction; throw it again.
6. Repeat until no air bubbles remain. Wedged clay should be used for all clay projects.

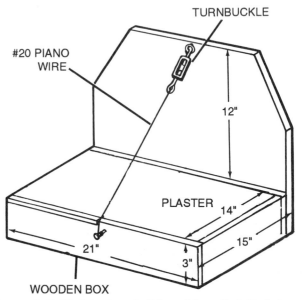

Figure 6–7. Wedging board. (Adapted from Craft Techniques in Occupational Therapy. Department of the Army, Washington, DC, 1980, p 3–12.)

Wedging clay is a repetitive task that requires bi-lateral coordination, strength, and endurance. It can be done in a sitting or standing position.

Pinch Pot

You will need:

Clay
Elephant ear sponge
Kemper tool
Turntable

1. Form a ball of clay 2 to 4 inches in diameter, depending on the size of the project you will be constructing.

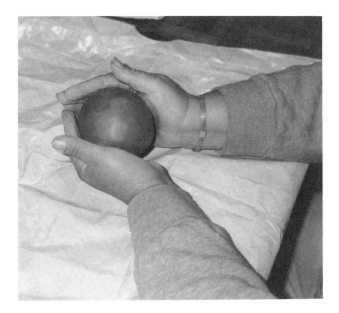

2. As you work, keep the clay moist by occasionally drizzling water onto it.
3. Depress the center of the ball with your thumbs, keeping the outside of the pot smooth.

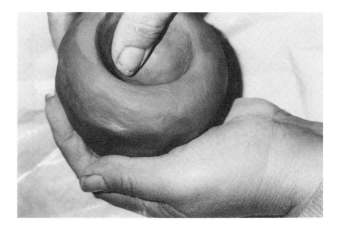

4. Rotate the pot as you work, pressing firmly and evenly into the clay. Increase the opening, thinning the walls to approximately ⅜ inch.
5. When your pot is the shape you like, smooth it with a damp sponge.

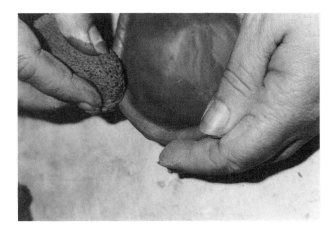

6. Trim the top edge evenly.
7. If you like, use a sharp tool to incise the clay with a decorative design.
8. Allow the pot to dry before firing.

Coil Building with Template

You will need:

Cardboard
Pencil
Craft knife

Template

1. Make a full-size drawing on paper of the piece you plan to make.
2. Fold the drawing in half vertically and cut it out.
3. Trace the folded drawing onto a piece of cardboard. Cut the shape out of the cardboard.
4. The outer piece is the template. Use it to keep the pot even as you work.

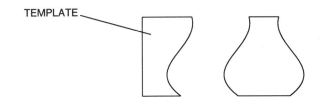

TEMPLATE

Pot

You will need:

Clay
Elephant ear sponge
Turntable

1. Flatten a ball of clay to ⅜ inch thickness for the base.

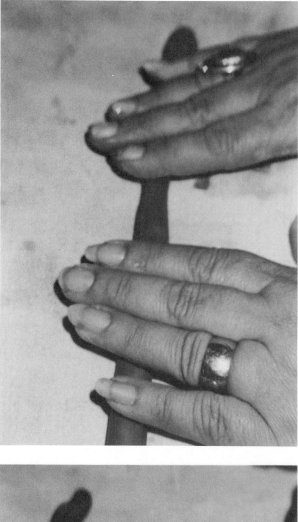

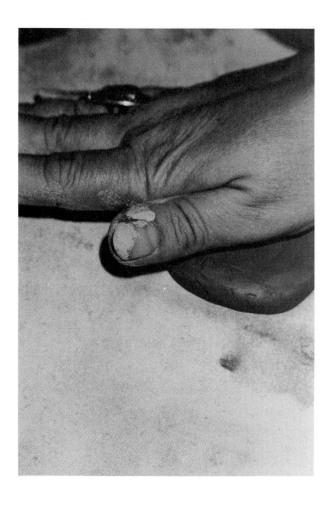

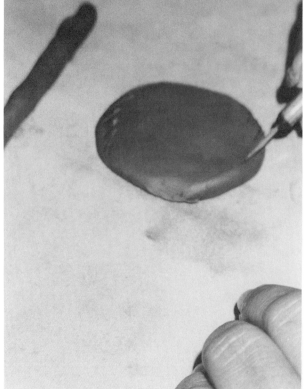

2. Working on a firm surface, form a coil approximately ½ inch in diameter, and 8 to 10 inches in length.
3. Roughen and moisten the clay surfaces where they touch.

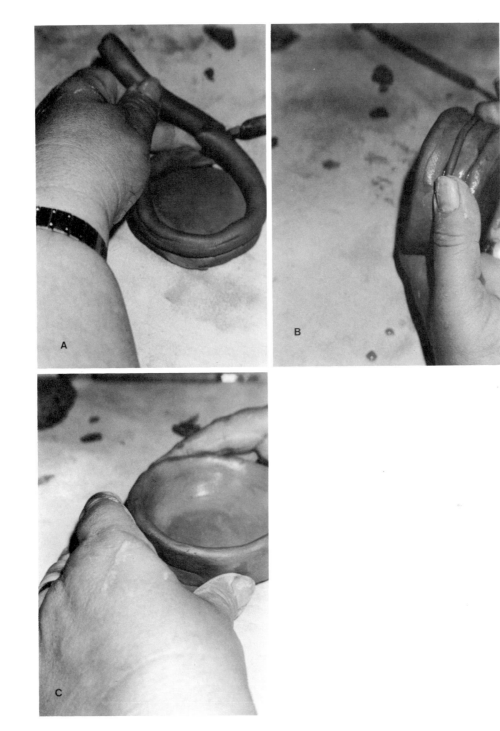

4. Cut the ends of the coil at an angle so that they will join without creating a bulge.

5. Wrap the coil atop the outer edge of the base.

6. Continue building upon the outer edge, turning and checking the pot against the template as you work until it is the shape and size you have designed.

7. Smooth the surface with a sponge or a straightedge.

8. Decorate the pot to your liking.

9. Allow to dry before firing.

Slab Construction

You will need:

Clay
Rolling pin
Pattern
Kemper tool
Elephant ear sponge

1. Place a ball of clay on a firm surface. Using a rolling pin or a glass jar or bottle, flatten the clay to an even thickness of ⅜ inch. Firing strips can be used to control the thickness.

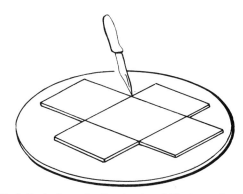

From Craft Techniques in Occupational Therapy. Department of the Army, Washington, DC, 1980, p 3-17.

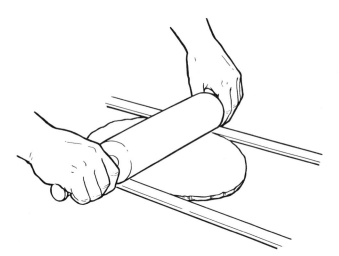

From Craft Techniques in Occupational Therapy. Department of the Army, Washington, DC, 1980, p 3-17.

2. The shape can be made free-form or from a pattern. Score around the pattern. Cut away the excess with a sharp tool.

3. Cut a 1-inch strip from a slab.
4. Wet and roughen the surfaces to be joined.
5. Press the strip against the base, working the joint so that it is smooth and even.
6. Finish with a sponge.
7. Allow to dry before firing.

Working clay is a bilateral task, requiring tactile discrimination. It may or may not require vision, but perception of space is necessary.

Wheel Throwing

Potter's wheels are usually operated by foot or knee pedals, by kicking, or by electricity.

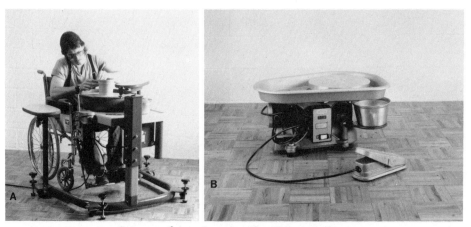

Courtesy of American Art Clay Company, Inc.

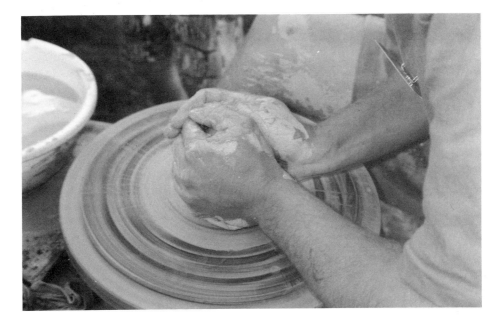

Kick wheels are more difficult to operate than other wheels because they require trunk control and coordination between the upper and lower extremities. They also require a good deal of space. Small portable electric wheels are commercially available and are generally more feasible for the clinic.

Centering is the most difficult phase of the process for the beginner to learn. Yet, like most skills, once you learn it, it's easy. It certainly appears easy when an experienced potter works, but throwing a pot requires considerable skill. If possible, have a potter show you how it's done. If you are adventurous, here's how to do it.

You will need:

Clay
Plaster bat
Wheel
Wire
Sponge

1. Center the bat by using slip to secure it to the wheel.
2. Place a ball of moist, wedged clay in the center of the bat.
3. As the wheel turns, with both hands on the clay, press down from the top and in from the sides toward the center of the wheel.
4. Moisten the clay as you work to keep it malleable.
5. Depress the center of the ball with the fingers.

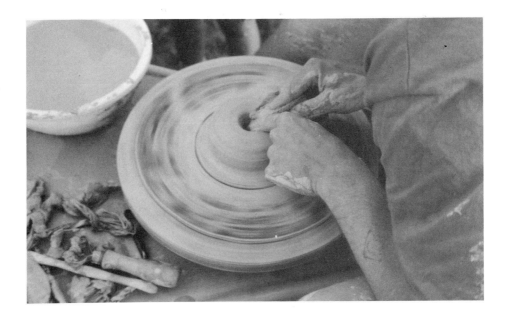

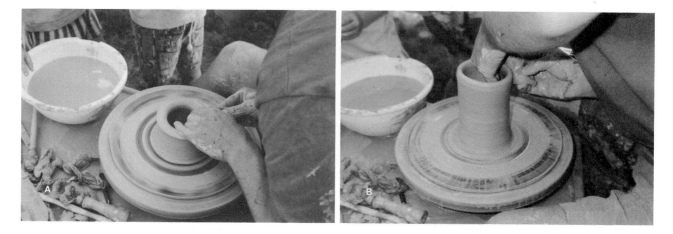

6. Draw up the sides of the pot by pressing on the inside and outside of the pot with the fingers of both hands.

7. When the pot is the size and shape you like, insert a wire at the top edge, cutting the excess off evenly as the pot turns.

8. Sponge finish.

9. Remove the pot from the bat by drawing a wire across the bottom while the wheel is turning.

10. Decorate as you prefer.

11. Allow to dry thoroughly before firing.

Preparing Greenware from Slip Molds

Slip is liquefied clay. Slip is poured into molds to produce items of identical form. Molds are made of plaster of paris and can be purchased commercially. Molds come in halves held together by bands.

You will need:

Plaster mold
Slip
Sandpaper
Glaze
Brush

1. Pour the slip into the mold; avoid forming air pockets.

2. Set the mold to dry. When dry, open the mold and remove the greenware.

3. Sand the greenware gently with fine sandpaper to remove the ridge where the mold halves come together.

4. Use a damp sponge to remove dust; otherwise, the glaze will not adhere.

5. Apply glaze with a brush.

6. Set aside to dry.

7. Fire.

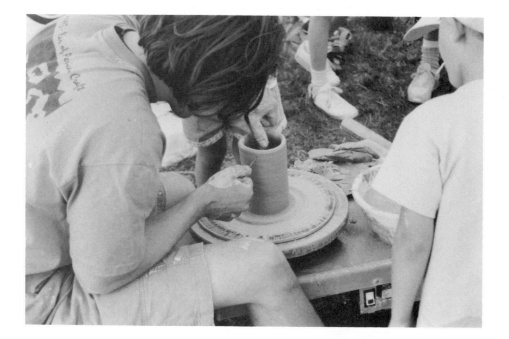

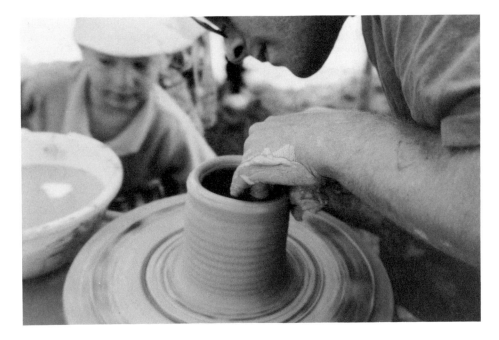

Items made from molds are very popular in clinics and generally assure an attractive product. They offer opportunities for choice, are simple to complete, require asymmetric hand use and some degree of eye-hand coordination, which varies depending on the size and complexity of the project. Preformed greenware and bisqueware can be purchased for the clinic, cutting down on preparation time in pouring molds and drying time. In some clinics, volunteers pour the molds.

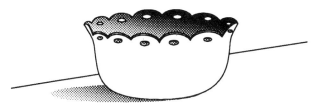

Figure 6–9. Excising. Portions of the clay are cut away, creating a design.

Ornamentation

1. **Incising.** Use a sharp tool to cut a design into the clay (Fig. 6–8).

2. **Excising.** Cut an area out of the walls of the pot, leaving a design (Fig. 6–9).

3. **Appliqué.** Form an ornamental shape out of clay. Scar the reverse side of the appliqué and the surface to which it will be applied. Moisten both surfaces and press the appliqué to the pot to form a raised design (Fig. 6–10).

4. **Glazing.** Glazing is used to color greenware or bisqueware or to provide a glasslike finish. Glazes come in matte and glossy finishes. Colored or clear glazes can be applied to greenware before firing. Bisqueware can also be glazed and refired. Refiring generally produces a finer and stronger product.

Potters often experiment with firing temperatures, clays, and glazes to obtain the effects they desire. Some are more than willing to share their findings; others zealously guard their secrets. Commercial glazes are reliable and will give you a good product, but trial and error make for the best learning. Follow manufacturers' directions.

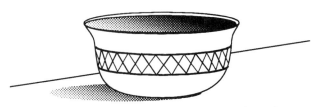

Figure 6–8. Incising. A tooler is used to inscribe a design in the clay before firing.

Figure 6–10. Appliqué. Pieces of clay are applied to a pot with slip, creating a raised design.

Glazed pots can be used to contain liquid; however, if the pots are to be used as containers for food or beverages, be absolutely certain of the safety of the glaze formulation. Glazes can leach into food, and some are toxic.

Firing

The oven in which clay is baked is called a kiln, pronounced "kill." Firing dried clay, called greenware, at extremely high temperatures (1000–2500°F) for extended periods (5–24 hours) transforms it into a hard ceramic material called bisque. Firing is also used to apply glazes. The production of ceramics depends on chemical reactions; therefore, differences in materials and temperatures produce varying effects (Table 6–1).

Table 6–1. FIRING TEMPERATURES

Cone	Celsius	Fahrenheit	Color of fire
15	1435	2615	
14	1400	2552	
13	1350	2462	
12	1335	2435	
11	1325	2417	
10	1305	2381	White
9	1285	2345	
8	1269	2300	
7	1250	2282	
6	1230	2246	
5	1205	2201	
4	1190	2174	
3	1170	2138	
2	1165	2129	
1	1160	2120	
01	1145	2093	Yellow
02	1125	2057	
03	1115	2039	
04	1060	1940	
05	1040	1904	
06	1015	1859	
07	990	1814	
08	950	1742	Orange
09	930	1706	
010	905	1661	
011	895	1643	
012	875	1607	Cherry red
013	860	1580	
014	830	1526	
015	805	1481	
016	795	1463	
017	770	1418	
018	720	1328	Dull red
019	660	1220	
020	650	1202	
021	615	1139	
022	605	1121	

Cones are used to monitor firing temperatures. Specific directions for firing depend on the kiln and materials being used. For best results, follow the manufacturers' instructions for loading and firing the kiln and for glazing.

Kilns require adequate space, insulation, and electrical wiring, although modern automatic kilns can be purchased in sizes that require much less space and no special wiring. Loading and operating a kiln requires time and attention not ordinarily available in the modern clinic. If volunteers are not available, it may be preferable to use other alternatives.

Sometimes outside potters are willing to fire pots if they are certain they are not likely to explode and damage other work. If you can find a potter who will cooperate with you, special arrangements can sometimes be made. Another practical solution is to use self-hardening clay.

Self-Hardening Clay

Self-hardening clay is a useful alternative to natural clay where space, time, and cost are factors. No costly kiln and space are necessary. Pinch, slab, and coil-built pots can be made of self-hardening clay, and special paints can be used to decorate them when they have dried. Fun projects can be produced; however, there is no comparison between this material and the quality and permanence of a ceramic pot that has been fired and glazed.

Nontoxic Modeling Dough

When using clay with children, preparing a dough recipe from household ingredients can be fun and safe.

Recipe 1

2 c. flour
2 Tbs. olive oil
Cold water
1 c. salt
Vegetable food coloring

Mix flour and salt. Slowly stir in water and oil. Squeeze until the clay feels smooth. Add coloring as desired. All ingredients can be put into a plastic bag that zips shut, mixed in the bag, and stored in the same bag for up to 1 week in the refrigerator.

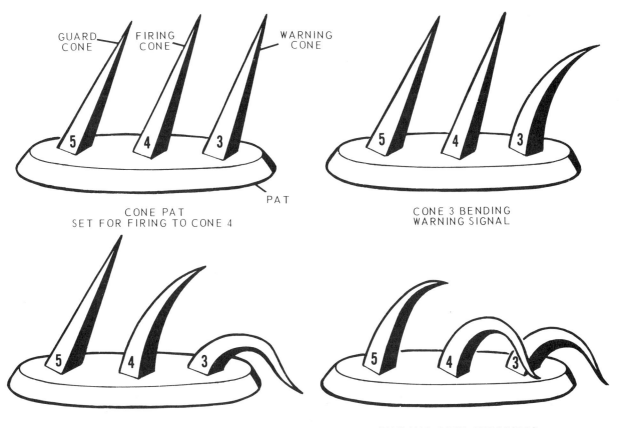

GUARD CONE   FIRING CONE   WARNING CONE

5   4   3

PAT

CONE PAT
SET FOR FIRING TO CONE 4

CONE 3 BENDING
WARNING SIGNAL

5   4   3

CONE 4 BENT-TIME TO TURN OFF KILN

KILN HAS BEEN OVERFIRED.

From Craft Techniques in Occupational Therapy. Department of the Army, Washington, DC, 1980, p 3-47.

Recipe 2

1 c. salt
½ c. boiling water
½ c. cornstarch
Vegetable food coloring

Stir salt, cornstarch, and water over low flame until stiff. Cool. Knead until pliable. Add vegetable coloring. Store in refrigerator.

Recipe 3

1 c. flour
1 c. water
1 Tbs. oil
½ c. salt
1 tsp. cream of tartar
Vegetable food coloring

Mix ingredients in a pan. Cook over medium heat until mixture pulls away from sides of pan and becomes dough. Knead until cool. This material is *not* edible. Keeps unrefrigerated for 3 months. Use over and over.

A commercial alternative to homemade dough is Play-Doh, which comes in bright and attractive colors that children find appealing.

MOSAICS

Times and Events

Mosaic tiles are glazed pieces of ceramic. These small bits of colored tile originally were used to decorate and protect walls, ceilings, and floors in and around the Mediterranean region. Ancient Babylonians, Egyptians, Greeks, and Romans developed mosaic decoration into a fine art. The beauty of their designs has endured for many hundreds of years. Tiles continue to be used throughout the modern world in bathrooms and other parts of the home and commercial establishments.

This craft of architectural origin was adapted into a leisure and fine-art activity. It often is used in the construction of trivets, ashtrays, murals, and other art pieces for which durability is of importance.

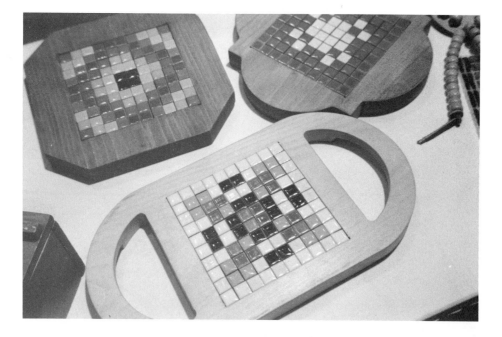

Tile comes in various colors and sizes. Those most commonly used for craft projects are ⅜-inch square, but tile can be found in other sizes. Craft tiles are usually attached to 12-inch-square sheets of loosely woven fabric. Individual tiles can be cut with a hand-gripped tile cutter to create interesting and well-fitted designs (Fig. 6–11).

For more interesting projects, one can make tiles by forming a slab of clay and cutting it into geometric shapes, then glazing and firing the pieces.

You will need:

Tiles
Water
Cement
Grout
Silicone polish
Tile cutter
Base

1. Soak the sheet of tiles until the tiles come loose from the fabric backing.
2. Set the tiles glazed-side-down onto paper towels or newspapers to dry.
3. Turn the tiles up and sort them by colors. Place into containers such as paper cups.
4. Select a base and plan your design. Use a tile cutter to fit the tiles into place.
5. Glue the tiles in place with cement, being sure to leave a ¹⁄₁₆-inch space between each tile.
6. Pour grout onto the surface of the tiles. Use a sponge to press the grout down between the tiles.
7. Sponge the excess grout off the surface of the tiles *before it dries* or it will harden and be impossible to remove.
8. After the grout dries, spray the tile surface with silicone polish. Shine with a soft cloth.

> Mosaic tile can be used for many clinical purposes. It can be an excellent assessment tool, revealing organizational abilities as well as fine motor skills. Tile cutting demands grasp strength.
>
> Be careful when cutting tile. Glaze is essentially glass. If fragments of tile fly up while it is being cut, eye or skin injuries can occur. To avoid accidents, be careful to cover the tile when cutting it, or wear goggles.

CASE EXAMPLES

Amy R., 38, has had multiple sclerosis for 12 years, exhibiting sporadic exacerbations and remissions throughout that period. Amy lives with her unmarried

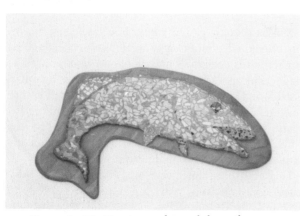

Figure 6–11. Mosaic on plywood, by author.

sister in a one-story home they inherited from their parents. During Amy's previous periods of remission she had been able to retain her job as a clerical worker. Since her last exacerbation, residual symptoms of incoordination and weakness in both upper extremities and blurred vision have increased to the point that she is no longer able to work at her clerical position.

Initial evaluation revealed intact 2-point discrimination in both upper extremities, grasp strength of 12 lbs on left, 17 lbs on right, with mild intention tremors. Sitting endurance is limited. The muscle power in her lower extremities is fair, and her balance is impaired. Visual deficits interfere with her ability to perform precise activities. Amy's sister is concerned about how Amy will adjust to her new forced retirement lifestyle at home.

GOALS

1. Increase strength and coordination in both upper extremities.
2. Increase tactile awareness to substitute for visual deficits.
3. Provide opportunities for developing leisure skills.

ACTIVITIES

Slab pot, pinch pot, coil pot, sand and glaze molded figurines.

As an outpatient, Amy was introduced to clay as a medium that would offer her a chance to exercise and strengthen her hands while developing a leisure skill. She was able to work the clay with her limited vision because her tactile sensitivity was sufficient to feel the pots. Amy began with coil-built pots, which allowed her to work smaller, less-resistant pieces. As she became more adept, she became quite interested in clay and joined a ceramics class in the local high school where she could have her work fired. She found she enjoyed sanding and glazing and began to experiment with new textured glazing techniques. Some of her work was exhibited in the local library and received commendation in the town art show. Although Amy continued to have exacerbations, she was able to continue with the ceramics during periods of remission.

Jack W., age 20, has been mentally retarded since birth. He lives in a group home and attends a program in a day training school. He is involved in a transitional school-to-work program, in preparation for working in a sheltered workshop. He exhibits limitations in attention span, fine motor performance, sequencing, and sorting skills. He has been assigned to an assembly-line task for training.

GOALS

1. Improve fine motor skills.
2. Improve work tolerance.
3. Develop appropriate work habits.

ACTIVITIES

Soak, turn, sort tiles in assembly line.

Jack spent 1 to 3 months at each workstation learning to soak and remove, turn the tiles face up, and sort the tiles by color. During these activities he was expected to display good work habits, such as being on time, being accurate, getting along with coworkers, being appropriate in interactions, and following supervisor's instructions. He was successful in these efforts and was referred to the State Division of Vocational Rehabilitation when he aged out of the school program at age 21.

BEADS

Times and Events

Beads have been found in every culture around the world from ancient to modern times (Fig. 6–12). They have been made of virtually every material. Consequently, because of their universal appeal and fundamental role in societies, they have been included here in one unit.

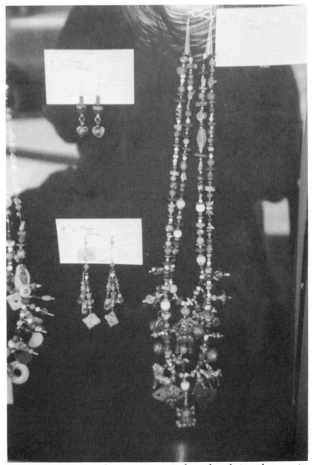

Figure 6–12. North American Indian bead jewelry, artist unknown.

Used as body decoration, beads reflect the inherent desire of people to ornament themselves, expressing both identity with their group and their own individuality. Beads are often characteristic of the environments from which they come. Pearls from the Orient and glass from Venice are among the most famous sorts of beads. Beads have been made of animal teeth, wood, clay, stone, and modern materials such as plastic. Commercially manufactured beads can be made into ornamental objects of all sorts, but the most fun comes when you start with beads you have made yourself.

Uniformity is ordinarily required in the manufacture of beads, although different styles and colors of beads can be mixed. Beads are strung into necklaces according to individual designs. In the past, beads were articles of trade. Today, people wear bead necklaces of all sorts. Jewelers and artists have taken this art form to extraordinary heights. Exotic bead necklaces are evidence of wealth in modern societies as well as ancient ones.

> Making beads is a precise activity. Designing a necklace allows one to be creative, and yet structured. Making a necklace requires fine motor and sequencing skills. Wearing a necklace one has made offers an opportunity for self-expression and enhanced self-image.

Figure 6–13. Ceramic bead necklace fashioned after ancient Middle Eastern jewelry, by workers in Israeli sheltered workshop.

Clay Beads

You will need:

Clay
Wire or cocktail straws
Glaze or paints
Dental floss
Needle

1. Pinch small pieces of clay into uniform pieces. Form them into small balls or rodlike shapes. Experiment to determine the size your beads will be.
2. Pierce each bead with a pin or wire, or insert a cocktail straw in the wet bead and allow it to dry. If you use wire to make holes, be sure the gauge of the wire is great enough to allow a needle to pass through the hole so the bead can be strung.
3. Move the wire periodically so that it can be removed when the bead has dried. If you use straws, cut them even with the surface of the beads when they are dry, leaving a plastic channel for the string.
4. Glaze and fire, or paint the bead with clay paints and finish with a glossy acrylic (Fig. 6–13).

Paper Beads

You will need:

Colored newsprint
Scissors
Toothpicks
Dental floss
Glue
Acrylic spray
Needle

1. Cut colored comics into triangles, approximately 1 inch at the base, and 6 inches in length.
2. Place a round toothpick along the 1-inch dimension and begin rolling the paper around the toothpick until the entire triangle is wound evenly and completely.
3. Secure the end with a dot of glue.
4. Slip the toothpick out. This will leave a hole that can be strung.
5. Spray the bead with acrylic.

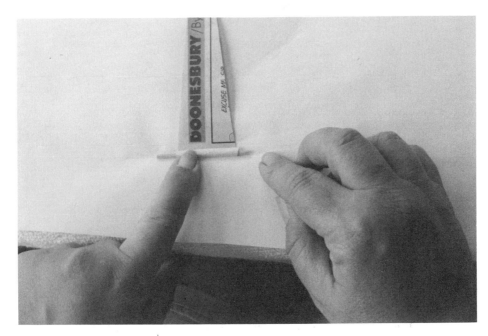

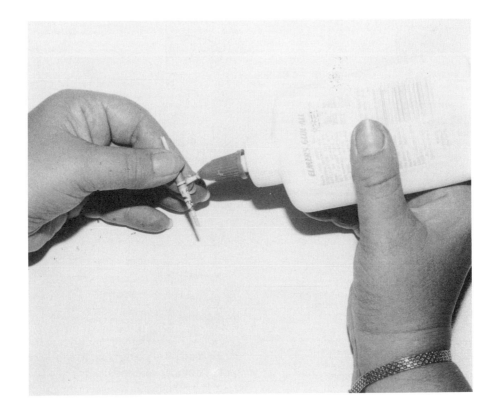

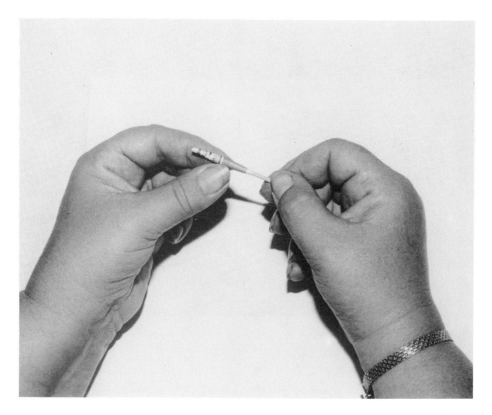

To vary the size of the beads, adjust the size of the paper triangles. To achieve other effects, different papers can be used, and the beads can be painted.

Stringing Beads

Necklaces are ordinarily symmetric, but they can be designed in any pattern and of many different shapes of beads. Attractive jewelry can be made by combining commercial beads with handcrafted ones (Table 6–2).

Table 6–2. COLORS OF STONES

Color	Stones
White	Pearls, rock crystal
Pink	Coral
Dark pink	Rose quartz, coral
Red	Ruby, coral
Maroon	Garnet
Yellow	Light amber, tigereye
Rust	Amber, carnelian
Dark blue	Lapis lazuli
Lilac	Amethyst
Violet	Amethyst
Bright green	Peridot, malachite
Light green	Jade
Beige	Pearls, amber, carnelian
Brown	Tigereye
Gray	Gray pearls, hematite
Black	Onyx, black pearls, obsidian

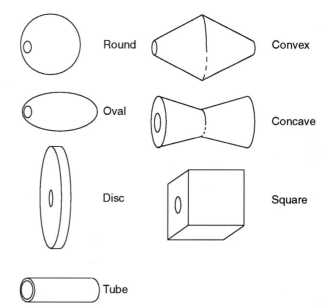

You will need:

Beads
Beading needle
Beading thread

1. Design a pattern in which both sides contain the same number of beads.

2. Lay the beads out according to the pattern you have designed. For irregularly sized beads, place them in pairs closest in size, arranging them so that the larger beads

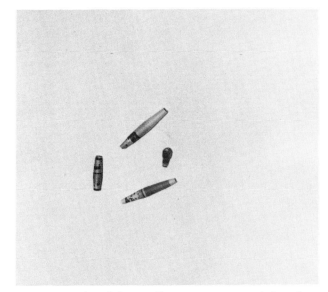

are at one end and the smaller ones are toward the other. Then divide the beads into two parallel groups.

3. Add one bead in the center that is larger than the others. This bead can be different from the others and makes a point of interest.

4. String the beads onto button thread, dental floss, or cord, tying the ends of the string to a ring. Precious beads are knotted individually and secured with a safety clasp.

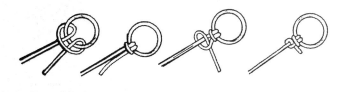

CASE EXAMPLE

Lillie L., 17, is in her junior year of high school and attends a center city rehabilitation program for substance abusers. She is uncooperative, easily distracted, competitive, occasionally self-abusive, and has low self-esteem. She states that she has no future. Her potential for future employment is dim because her interpersonal skills would limit her at any job. Her only interests seem to be in fashion.

GOALS

1. Increase self-esteem.
2. Improve concentration, work tolerance, and other prevocational skills.
3. Develop interpersonal skills through peer group activities.

ACTIVITIES

Design and create jewelry in group environment.

Lillie was encouraged to join a group that designs and creates jewelry that is marketed through the clinic consignment shop. Precision and productivity are required in bead making and assembly. The group sets the standards for production and payment is calculated accordingly. Bonuses are awarded for new design ideas. Lillie's interest in fashion design and her competitiveness stimulated her interest and ability in designing necklaces. Workers who are judged reliable by their peers are permitted to work in the store, where additional income can be earned. Lillie's competitive nature was helpful in improving her cooperation in the production group. As her behavior improved, the group voted her privileges in the shop, where she was found to be a successful salesperson, ultimately working her way up to store manager. Once discharged from the program, she was able to use the skills she acquired to obtain a retail position in a costume jewelry shop. She now volunteers at the rehabilitation program regularly.

BASKETS

Times and Events

Baskets were among the earliest tools people used to carry and store things of value (Fig. 6–14). Some historians believe that birds' nests were the earliest baskets, and that these nests served as models for the ones ancient peoples learned to make. Learning from their world, ancient peoples used their creativity and dexterity to adapt materials for personal needs.

The many different natural materials from which baskets are made reflect the environments from which they come. Baskets were made of materials that grew locally. They have been constructed of grasses, reeds, vines, and even the needles of pine trees. Cultures can be identified by the materials and designs of their baskets. Because baskets are composed of degradable materials, few truly ancient examples remain. However, some modern cultures still use basketry in the same ways that ancient peoples did.

Baskets are as popular today as ever, both as implements and as art forms. Made of many different materials, baskets are designed to meet special uses. Among the many kinds of ancient and modern baskets are creels for fish, trays for cut flowers, and baskets for harvesting and for laundry (Figs. 6–15 and 6–16).

Modern artists continue to create lovely items from natural materials that are freely available today from around the world through trade and transportation (Fig. 6–17). They also use synthetic materials in their designs. Modern baskets, while artistic, may or may not be utilitarian. To add interest to a basket's design, reed can be dyed and spray-painted. Some basketweavers include unusual materials in their baskets for design interest.

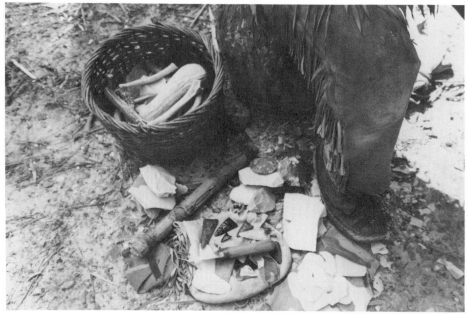

Figure 6-14. Basket holding flint knapper tools.

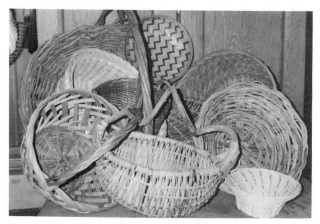

Figure 6-15. Assorted baskets.

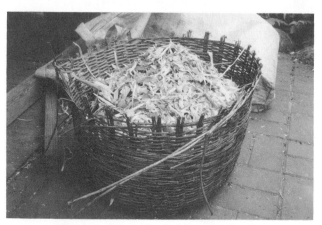

Figure 6-16. Basket holding wood chips.

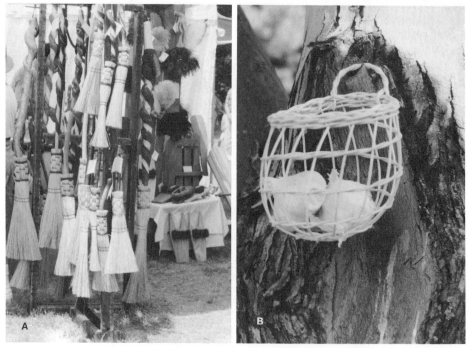

Figure 6-17. (*A*) Straw brooms. (*B*) Garlic basket.

> Be cautious about using basketry with patients who have skin disorders, as working with damp reed can be irritating to the skin. Some materials splinter and can cause injury.

Reed and Wood Basket

The wooden base is an adaptation designed to make a basket easy to construct, especially for beginners, because it holds the reeds in place (Fig. 6–18). Round or oval wooden bases are commercially available but can be made easily from plywood by drilling an uneven number of holes equal distances apart in each base.

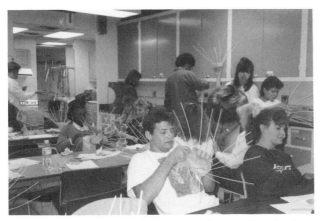

Figure 6–18. Occupational therapy students making baskets.

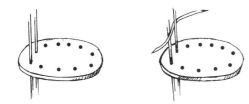

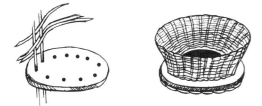

You will need:

Reed, #2, #4. The higher the number, the thicker the reed.
Wooden base
Clippers
Fid
Water pail

1. Cut sufficient spokes of #4 reed, 18 inches in length, for the number of holes in the base.
2. Soak the reed in water for approximately 15 minutes until it is flexible; do not soak it longer than necessary, or it will fray.
3. Insert a spoke into each hole, extending 15 inches above and 2½ inches below each hole.
4. Work on the underside first, holding the base so that the edge of the wood faces you.
5. Starting at any point, lay the first reed in front of one immediately to its right, and behind the next. Continue until all the ends are woven firmly.
6. Secure the last reed in front of the one you started with and behind the next one to its right. If you have done this correctly, you will not be able to tell where you began.
7. Turn the basket over so the long spokes face up.
8. Select a long weaver of #2 reed and weave alternately behind and in front of each spoke. Press down firmly against the base as your work. The shape of the basket is governed by tension from the weaver. You can create interesting shapes by pulling the reed more or less taut. Do not pull in too tightly as you weave or the basket will assume a shape you may not like. Beginners should strive for uniform or symmetrical forms until they become skilled.
9. As the weaving progresses, you will need to start a new weaver. Overlap the old and new weavers on the inside of the basket, across a spoke.
10. When the basket has assumed the desired height, cut the weaver with the clippers.

Finishing

A basket can be finished in a number of ways. One attractive and easy method is as follows:

1. Place one spoke in front of two spokes to its right and behind the next one. Continue in this way around the basket. Finish in keeping with the same pattern.
2. Trim the ends at an angle. Be careful not to cut them too short, or they may come loose.

Reed Basket

Traditional baskets are made entirely of reed. They are more difficult to construct than wooden base baskets but preceded them historically.

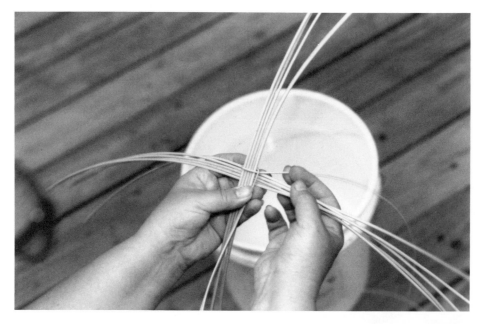

You will need:

Reed   Fid
Clippers   Water pail

1. As always when constructing a basket, keep the reed moist by periodically soaking it in a pail of water.

2. Cut ten 15-inch lengths of #4 reed to form the spokes. Place the reeds into two groups of 5. Cross one group of reeds over the other at the center as shown.

3. Select a long weaver. Bend it into two parallel strands of unequal length, so the splices will not be in the same place.

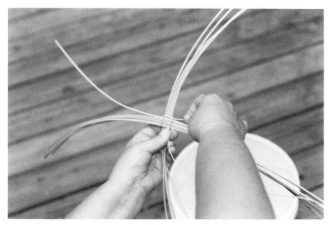

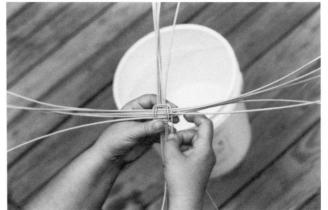

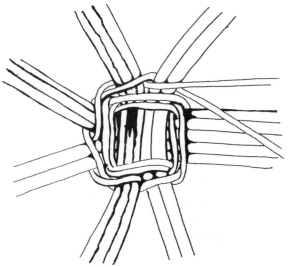

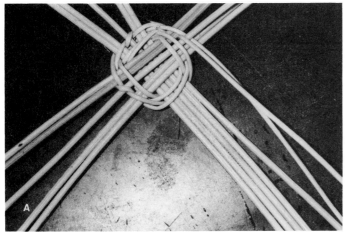

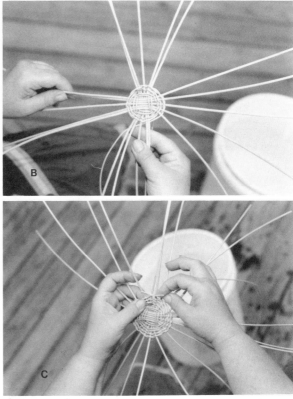

4. Wrap the weaver around one group of 5 spokes. Twist the strands, reversing their top and bottom positions over the next group of 5 spokes; twist again. Continue in this way 2 times around, always twisting in the same direction.

5. Break down each group of 5 spokes to groups of 2, 1, and 2 by twisting the weaver between the groups. Go around 2 times.

6. Break down into individual spokes, twisting the weavers between each spoke. Continue weaving until the base is 3 to 4 inches wide. Add additional weavers as needed.

7. Being sure the spokes are damp, turn them up at 90° angles. Continue to weave, shaping the basket.

8. Finish the edge using the same technique described for the wooden base basket. Many other finishing techniques are also possible. Investigate how other baskets are made and finished, and experiment.

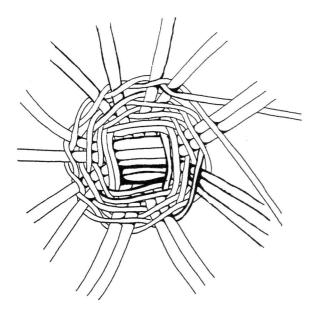

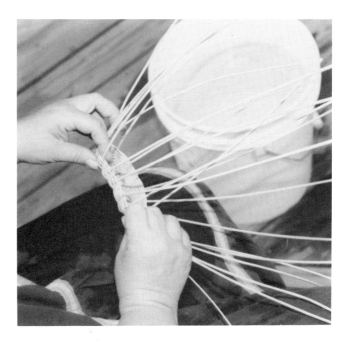

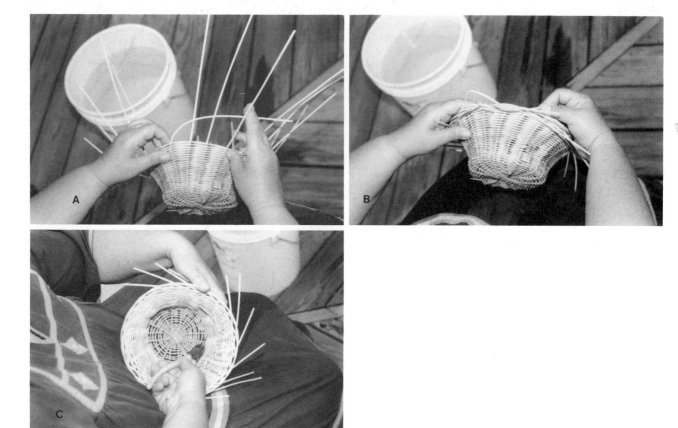

Vine Basket and Wreath

The fun of making a vine basket or wreath starts when you collect your materials. Natural materials can be found in rural areas. Wild grape vines have curly projections that add interest to a finished basket. Wisteria, honeysuckle, and morning glory have different qualities and also make attractive baskets.

Be familiar with wilderness plants; be careful not to pick poisonous or endangered species. Wear gloves to protect your hands, and use clippers. Always get permission before picking. Many people will be delighted to

have you ask, but do not cut just any part of the vine haphazardly. Ask if there is a particular way to cut the vine. Vines tend to choke out gardens, so essentially you will be doing a much needed weeding job.

When constructing a vine basket, you can use one or several materials. If you use more than one type of material, use the heavier ones for the spokes and the lighter ones as the weaver. Weave and finish the edge the same way the reed basket is done, or create a design of your own. Vine baskets look particularly beautiful with dried wildflowers or herbs in them. To make a wreath, simply wrap the vine in a circle and hang to dry.

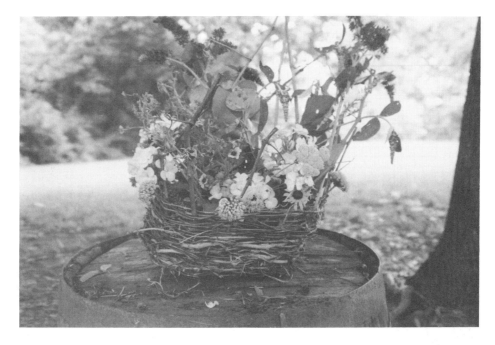

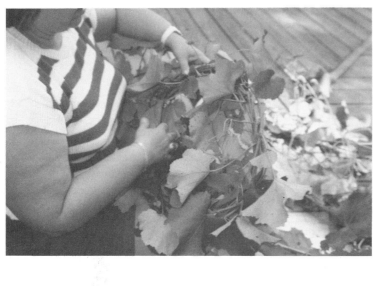

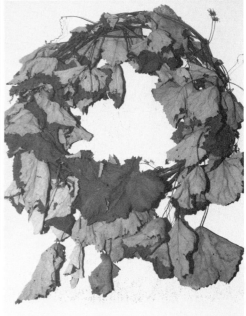

CASE EXAMPLE

Marvin M., 27, a press operator, sustained a crush injury to the second, third, and fourth fingers of his dominant right hand. Surgical reductions of fractures of the middle finger and tendon surgery of the forefinger were performed. Following surgery, the hand was immobilized for 3 weeks, after which time therapy began. Marvin had residual deficits in flexion and extension of the second, third, and fourth fingers of the right hand and limitations in grasp strength and dexterity.

GOALS

1. Increase flexion and extension of the proximal and distal joints of the second, third, and fourth fingers of the right hand.

2. Increase grasp strength and dexterity in the right hand to functional levels.

3. Improve bilateral coordination.

4. Return to former employment.

ACTIVITY

Begin with wooden-base basket and upgrade to reed basket as skills improve.

Marvin was given a choice of several activities that would allow him to meet the goals established for his recovery. He selected basketry because his roommate collected baskets and this would be a gift. Marvin was instructed to wear a rubber glove to protect the incisions from water. When he completed the first basket, the therapist suggested he try to make a reed basket that required more dexterity and strength and would give him more practice. Instead, Marvin brought some grape vines and honeysuckle from his backyard into the clinic and made a beautiful vine basket. Marvin gained sufficient grasp strength, dexterity, and bilateral coordination in his right hand to return to work 4 months after the accident.

LEATHER

Times and Events

Leather is a durable material that has been used for clothing and shelter since earliest times. It continues to be used today for many functional and ornamental purposes. Leather is made from animal skins that have been tanned to preserve them. Cowhide, kidskin, snake skin, eelskin, and other materials are popular leathers. Manufacturers often take steer hide and process it to look like other leathers. Synthetic materials can be used in the same way as natural leathers. These modern materials are very popular because they protect endangered species of animals. Modern designers use these remarkable materials to make appealing and salable items.

> Leathers are attractive, versatile materials that offer many opportunities for creative expression, while requiring precise workmanship.

Making a Pattern

A good first project is a case for something you keep in your pocket, such as scissors, comb, pocketknife, pen and pencil, business cards, or eyeglasses.

You will need:

Cardboard
Scissors or craft knife
Rule
Pencil
Paper

1. Select an item that needs a leather case.
2. Trace the item on paper.

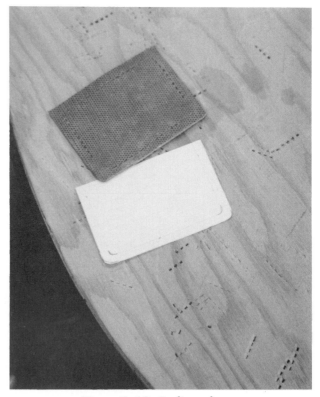

Figure 6–19. Credit card case.

3. Add ¼ inch all around the tracing (Fig. 6–19). Allow extra width on the pattern for items of depth such as eyeglasses.
4. Cut out the pattern. Before proceeding further, be certain to check the size of the pattern against the item.

If your project has a front and back that differ somewhat, such as a container with a flap, cut 2 patterns. Be certain they are identical in size, with the exception of any details that differ.

Leather Case

You will need:

Leather
Pattern
Tooler
Steel rule
Craft knife
Utility shears
Rubber cement

1. Select a piece of leather large enough and of the correct quality for the project you have designed. Shoe leather differs markedly from glove leather, as they serve different needs. Be sure to select leather suitable for your project.

2. Leather is costly, so conserve the material. Lay the pattern against the leather's edge, making as little waste as possible. However, be careful to avoid any blemishes in the leather. Remember, your project will have a front and a back, so plan accordingly for the size leather you need. Ordinarily, several projects can be cut from one skin. Use scrap leather for small projects.

3. Press firmly around the pattern with the pointed end of a tooler so that an impression appears in the leather. This may be done on the rough side of the leather.

4. Using a steel rule as a straightedge, cut on the line with a sharp knife; cut freehand with utility shears for curves.

5. Repeat for the second half of the project.

6. Place both halves of the project together to be sure they fit. Trim if necessary, but do not cut away too much or your case will not fit the object for which you are making it.

7. Put rubber cement on the rough side of three edges of both sides of the project, taking care not to glue the opening shut. Allow the cement to become sticky. Press both pieces of leather together. Rubber cement can be pulled apart and reset without a problem.

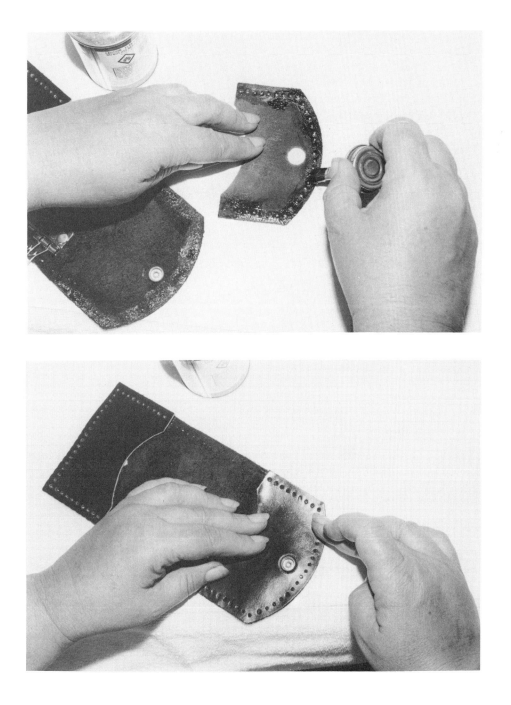

Use caution in the use of sharp tools. However, keep in mind that patients have access to tools when at home. Denying them their use may not be as effective as teaching them safe methods of use, and confidence in their use, while in a supervised environment. Also, note that sharp tools are safer to use than dull tools because they are less apt to slip.

Rubber cement should be used in a well-ventilated area.

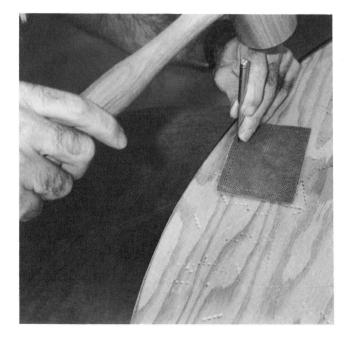

Hole Punching

Three kinds of tools are customarily used to make holes in leather: slit punch, rotary or single-hole punch, and awl. Slit punches and hole punches are used for leather lacing. The slit punch leaves a finer finish than a hole punch and is preferred by master leathercrafters. Awls are used for saddle stitching. A mallet is used with the slit punches and awl.

Slit Punch

Slit punches have one to six prongs. A one-prong punch and a four-prong punch are adequate for most leatherwork.

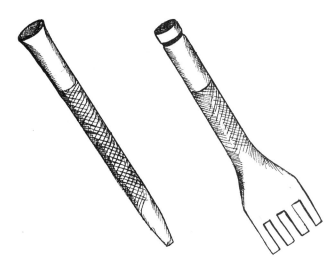

1. Mark a line ⅜ inch from the outer border using a steel rule and a tooler.
2. Place the four-prong slit punch on the line, beginning ⅜ inch from one corner of the leather.
3. Tap firmly with a mallet so that the punch goes through both pieces of leather at once.

4. Move the slit punch along the line, setting one prong of the punch into the last hole punched to keep the spacing even.
5. Use the single punch to make holes in corners or on curved edges. When using a single-prong punch be careful to retain equal distances between slits.

Using a slit punch demands concentration, precision, and bilateral hand function.

Rotary or Hole Punch

Precut key cases, coin purses, and wallets are punched with rotary or hole punches (Fig. 6–20). These items also can be used as patterns for projects of your own making.

1. Mark a line ⅜ inch from the outer border.
2. Set the rotary punch to the width of the lacing.
3. Place the punch on the mark and punch through both pieces of leather each time.

Using a hole punch demands grasp strength and endurance. Varying the size of the holes allows you to grade the resistance and therefore the strength needed to pull the lace through the holes.

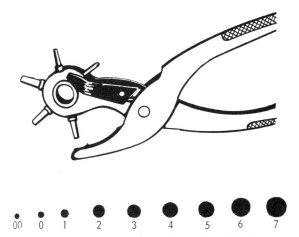

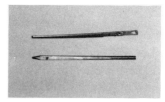

Figure 6–20. Rotary punch with graduated tube sizes. (Adapted from Craft Techniques in Occupational Therapy. Department of the Army, Washington, DC, 1980, p 11-13.)

Awl

The awl is used to pierce the leather for saddle stitching.

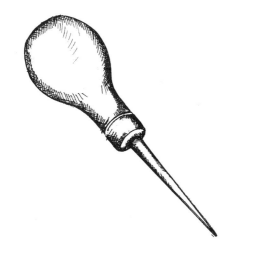

1. Mark the leather every ¼ inch around three sides of the project only, as the opening will not be stitched.
2. Place the leather onto a wooden surface.
3. Place the point of the awl on the mark, and use a mallet to hit the awl.
4. Repeat until all the holes are made.

> Awls are particularly sharp and potentially dangerous. Place a cork on the point when it is not in use.

Leather Lacing

Leather lacing can be done with or without a needle. Although some leathercrafters work without one, using a needle is easier and is recommended. Keep a tooler or fid handy to stretch the holes. Leather is resilient and will return to its original size if not dampened.

Leather needles are of several designs. One is like a tip on a shoelace. Another type is secured to the lacing by tapping the end closed with a mallet. One type is secured by twisting the pointed end of the lacing into a hole at the top of the needle. When finished, untwist to remove any remaining lace.

Three of the most commonly used leather lacing stitches are described in order of their increasing complexity:

You will need:

Leather project
Leather lacing
Leather needle
Tooler or fid
Duco cement
Skiver or knife

Whip Stitch

The whip stitch is the simplest leather lacing stitch. Measure 4 times the distance around the project to determine the amount of lacing required. Tuck the beginning of the lace between the 2 pieces of leather and pull through. Then simply insert the lacing into each succeeding hole from front to back, wrapping around to partially cover the edges. Be careful to keep the lacing from twisting. Finish by tucking the end under the lacing.

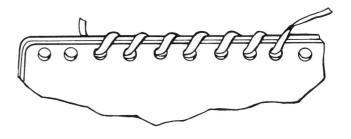

Single Cordovan

The single cordovan stitch is like a buttonhole stitch in embroidery.

1. Measure 5½ times the distance around the project to determine the amount of lacing required.

2. There is a front and a back to the stitch. Determine which is the face or front of the piece and keep it toward you as you work. Begin where there will be little wear and tear, not at a corner, unless the design requires starting there. Keep the lacing untwisted and taut as you work.

3. Stitch from left to right. *Insert the lacing into the hole from front to back. Repeat in the next hole to the right. Insert the lace into the loop that has formed at the top edge of the leather,** keeping the lacing on the left side of the loop for a consistent appearance. Repeat from * to ** around three sides of the project.

4. When you come to the corners, stitch 2 times in each corner hole to keep the lacing even.

5. When you come to the end of a piece of lacing, splice on another piece. Skive (shave) the top surface of the old lace and the bottom surface of the new lace approximately ⅜ inch from the ends. Glue these ends together with Duco cement. Allow to dry (Fig. 6–21).

6. On the 4th side, leave an opening by lacing only through 1 piece of leather.

7. Lace the remaining side of the opening with a

FINISHING. This stitch can be finished invisibly on projects in which the lacing circumvents the entire piece.

1. Slip the lace out of the first stitch leaving a loop.

2. Insert the end of the lace through the loop and back through the last loop.

3. Pull the first stitch out of the first hole. Insert the lace through the hole.

4. On the reverse side, trim the ends to ⅜ inch.

5. Skive the top surface of one end of the lace and the bottom of the other. Glue with Duco cement. If done properly, no seam will show.

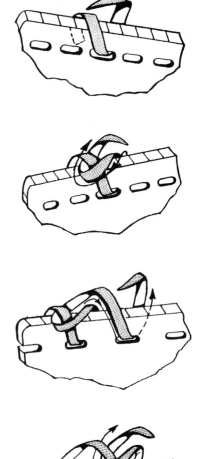

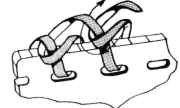

From Craft Techniques in Occupational Therapy. Department of the Army, Washington, DC, 1980, p 11-40.

Double Cordovan

The double cordovan is the most complex and ornamental of the lacing stitches described here.

1. Measure 7 times the distance around the project to determine the amount of lace you will need. Begin where there will be little wear and tear, not at a corner, unless the design of the project requires starting there.

2. This stitch has a right and a wrong side. Face the front of the piece toward you as you work. Always work from front to back, being certain to keep the lacing untwisted at all times.

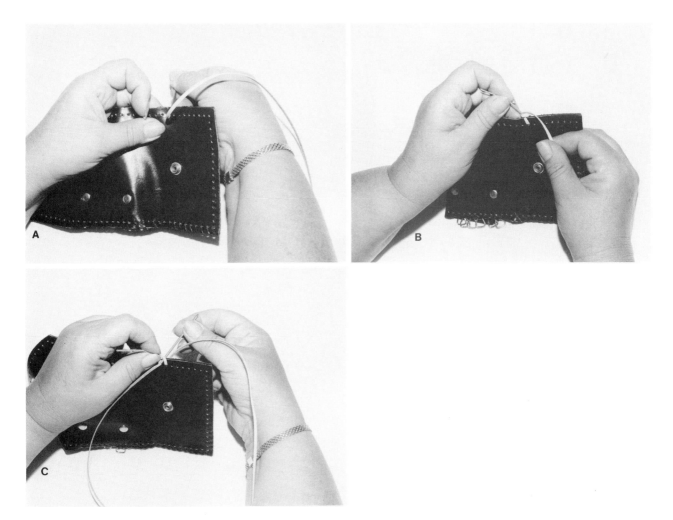

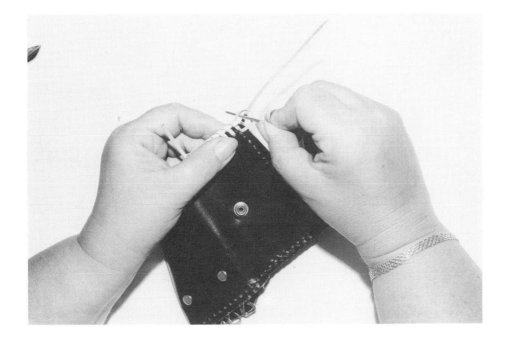

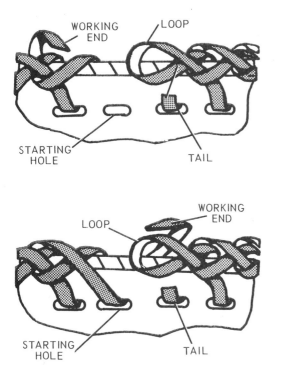

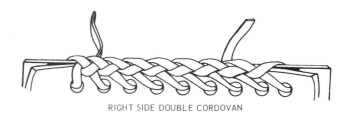

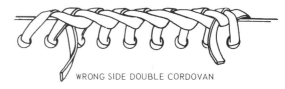

RIGHT SIDE DOUBLE CORDOVAN

WRONG SIDE DOUBLE CORDOVAN

From Craft Techniques in Occupational Therapy. Department of the Army, Washington, DC, 1980, p 11-40.

From Craft Techniques in Occupational Therapy. Department of the Army, Washington, DC, 1980, p 11-49.

3. Insert the lacing into the first hole.
4. Enter the next hole.
5. Insert the lacing into the loop on top.
6. Then *go into the next hole.
7. Lacing from front to back, go through the cross that has formed at the top.

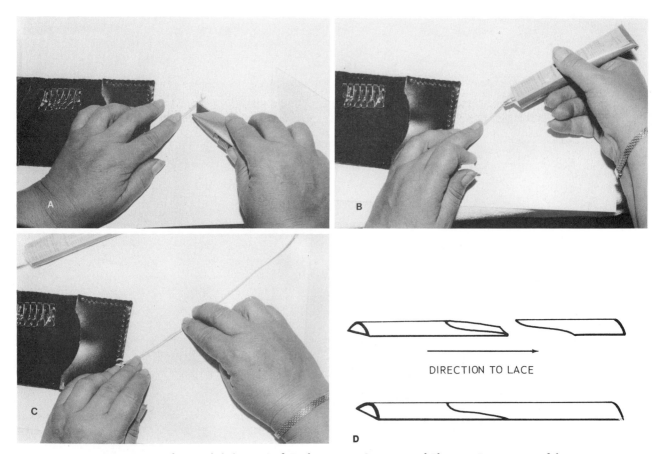

DIRECTION TO LACE

Figure 6–21. Skiving. (*D*) (From Craft Techniques in Occupational Therapy. Department of the Army, Washington, DC, 1980, p 11-41.)

8. Working from the back, pull the left loop taut, then pull the right loop taut.**

9. Repeat from * to ** all the way around.

10. At each corner, do two stitches into the same hole so that the lacing lies flat.

FINISHING. This stitch can be finished invisibly on projects in which the lacing circumvents the entire piece.

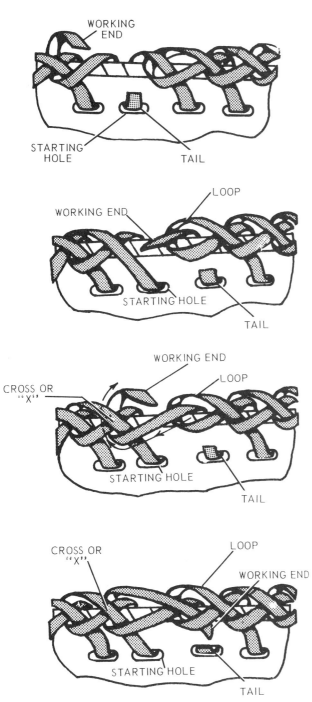

From Craft Techniques in Occupational Therapy. Department of the Army, Washington, DC, 1980, p 11-49.

1. Slip the beginning stitch out of the first loop and out of the first hole, leaving the loop intact.

2. Insert the end of the lace up through the first loop, through the last cross, down through the first loop, and into the remaining hole.

3. On the reverse side, trim the ends to ⅜ inch.

4. Skive the top surface of one end of the lace and the bottom of the other.

5. Glue one over the other with Duco cement, tucking the end under the stitching. If done properly, no seam will show.

Saddle Stitching

Saddle stitching gives the work a tailored appearance. As its name suggests, saddle stitching is used for making livery and saddle bags, but it is often seen on elegant handbags, sandals, and belts. Both sides of the work are identical.

You will need:

Two blunt tapestry needles
Button thread
Beeswax
Scissors

1. Place the project (Figs. 6–22 and 6–23) into a vise so that the holes are visible.

2. Measure a length of thread 2½ times the distance around the project. Thread 2 blunt-tipped heavy-gauged needles with waxed button thread.

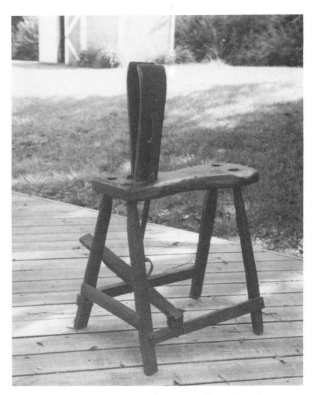

Figure 6–22. Antique harnessmaker's bench.

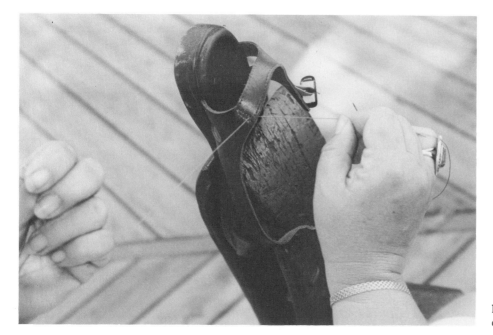

Figure 6–23. Repairing torn sandal using saddle stitching.

3. Position the work so that it is centered in front of you.

4. Insert one needle into the first hole. Pull through, leaving equal lengths of thread on each side.

5. As you work, rub beeswax along the thread. This will strengthen the thread and aid in pulling it through the leather.

6. Insert both needles into the next hole from opposite directions.

7. Exchange the needles into the opposite hands and pull taut.

8. Repeat the process around all 3 sides, leaving the opening unstitched.

9. Finish by reversing direction into the last 2 stitches.

10. Cut the threads snugly against the surface of the leather.

Saddle stitching is a resistive bilateral activity requiring fine and gross coordination.

Tooling

Tooling (Fig. 6–24) is an attractive and inexpensive way to decorate leather. A bookmark is a simple and useful project for learning this technique.

You will need:

Pattern
Tooling leather
Newspaper
Sponge
Water
Tooler
Paper towel

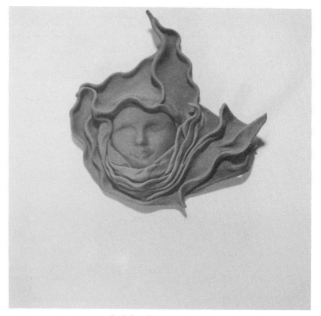

Figure 6–24. Tooled leather sculpture, artist unknown.

1. Draw a rectangle 1½ × 7 inches on paper.

2. Create a design within the rectangle. Flowers, leaves, initials, and other simple motifs are good design ideas. Keep the design open without too much detail. Children's coloring books are good sources for designs of this sort.

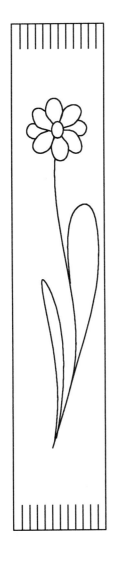

3. Cut a piece of thin, flexible tooling leather to the same dimensions as your pattern.

4. Secure your design to the leather with masking tape.

5. Work on a hard, smooth surface. Use the pointed end of a tooler to mark the design's outline onto the leather. This can be done on the rough side of the leather. Before removing the paper pattern, be certain your impression has come through onto the leather.

6. Prepare a thick (approximately 1 inch) pile of newspapers for the next step.

7. Place the leather face down onto the newspaper.

8. If you are using light-colored leather, place a piece of paper towel between the leather and the newspaper to keep the leather from becoming soiled with newsprint.

9. Dampen the leather with a moist sponge, taking care not to saturate the leather.

10. With the blunt end of the tooler, press heavily in the areas you want raised.

11. Turn the project face up.

12. Return the leather to the firm surface and depress the background.

13. Repeat the process until you are satisfied, dampening the leather as you work. You will have created a bas relief design.

14. The bookmark can be fringed if the design lends itself to this effect. Measuring carefully with a ruler, divide the width across the bottom into equal ¼-inch segments, 1 inch in length. Mark the lines for the fringes with a tooler. Cut carefully on the lines with a sharp craft knife and a steel rule.

> Leather tooling uses the same muscles used for handwriting and can be a good prewriting activity.

Stamping

Stamping is another way to ornament leather. This technique is similar to tooling but requires a special set of tools to create artistic designs in the leather. Once the leather is ornamented, it can be made into purses, belts, sandals, briefcases, and so on.

A coaster is a good project for beginners. Round blanks of leather are reasonably priced. They often come with paper designs, or you can make your own. Beginner sets are available that contain a small selection of tools.

You will need:

Steer hide
Stamping tools
Sponge

1. Dampen the leather.

2. Using a tooler, transfer the design from a paper pattern to the leather.

3. Using a special swivel knife designed for this purpose, score the design's outline onto the leather. Be careful not to cut too deeply, so you do not cut through the leather.

4. Select stamping tools to create the design.

5. Working with damp leather, tap the stamping tools with a wooden mallet to ornament the leather.

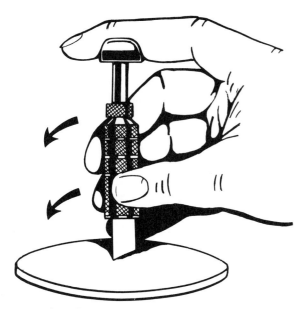

From Craft Techniques in Occupational Therapy. Department of the Army, Washington, DC, 1980, p 11-32.

Like tooling, leather carving uses the same muscles used for handwriting and can be a good prewriting activity. However, most projects of this sort require a considerable investment of time and effort. They are suitable leisure time activities and can even be a potential source of income. Well-crafted pieces are highly marketable.

Finishing

Leather can be dyed to add to its attractiveness. When dyed leather is cut, the raw edge reveals the original color of the leather. Dyeing the edge to match the surface improves the appearance of the project.

You will need:

Sandpaper
Leather dye
Leather polish
Soft cloth

1. Sand edges smooth.
2. Apply dye to the raw edges.
3. Allow to dry, then sand again and polish for a finished look.
4. Use a leather polish and buff to a sheen.

CASE EXAMPLE

John C., 24, a ranch hand, sustained a spinal cord injury at C7, in an automobile accident. He was left permanently nonambulatory, requiring a wheelchair. He had deficits in sitting balance and weakness in both upper extremities. Grasp was functional but weak because of the lack of strength and stability of the proximal musculature.

GOALS

1. Improve sitting tolerance and balance.
2. Increase upper-extremity strength.
3. Improve work tolerance.
4. Adjust to disability.
5. Expand leisure skills.

ACTIVITIES

Cutting, stamping, saddle stitching.

John was depressed following the accident. He had been an active horseman and recognized that he was never going to be able to resume that part of his life. During their initial conversation, the therapist began to focus on the job John had ahead of him in strengthening what he had left. She explored his interests and discovered his interest in horsemanship and the livery used in that occupation. He had admired that kind of work. She asked him if he knew how leatherwork was done. Then she showed him how to do stamping and told him he could try it. She adapted the tools by building up the handles to aid in grasp. After some practice on a coaster, John worked on a leather belt and became very adept. He tried saddle stitching using vise grips to give him additional power in grasping the needles. John became very good at leatherwork and as his work tolerance, balance, and strength improved, he developed a steady stream of customers for his work. John continued leatherwork as a leisure activity when he was discharged. He was referred to rehabilitation counseling for vocational testing and placement.

FIBERCRAFTS

Times and Events

Natural fibers are derived from plants and animals from around the world. Despite the fact that the flora and fauna differed from one environment to another, around the globe, people devised remarkably similar ways of using fibers to create cloth of all kinds: linen from flax, cotton from cotton plants, wool from sheep, silk from silkworms, cashmere from vicuna, and angora from rabbits. Furthermore, animals used for their fibers were not destroyed; instead, their fibers were harvested as a crop, suggesting an early awareness of the value of conservation.

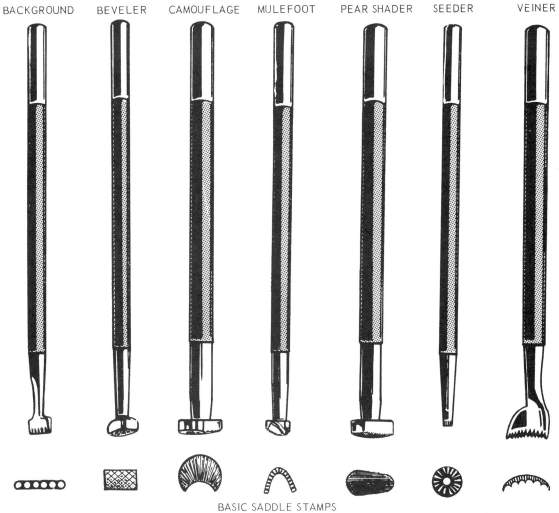

BACKGROUND   BEVELER   CAMOUFLAGE   MULEFOOT   PEAR SHADER   SEEDER   VEINER

BASIC SADDLE STAMPS

From Craft Techniques in Occupational Therapy. Department of the Army, Washington, DC, 1980, p 11-16.

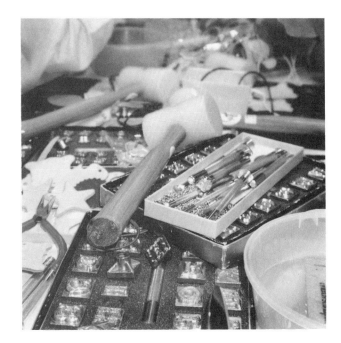

With the advent of the petrochemical industry, modern fibers were developed, expanding the diversity of materials available for the manufacturing of cloth. Nylon, rayon, Orlon, and polyester are some of these materials. Each can be spun into yarn and thread to be used for weaving and other needlecrafts.

Weaving techniques used for these different fibers are universal in concept and originated as adaptations of basketry. From ancient to modern times, the production of cloth developed according to degrees of mechanization from simple to complex looms. Methods of making objects from cloth were automated to increasing degrees with the development of electricity and then computerization.

Innumerable items can be made from yarn using many different yarncraft techniques. Regardless of the means of production, artistic designs have always been an element in the manufacturing of cloth and are evident in clothing and furnishings of all sorts. Yarn and cloth are virtually limitless in scope and design. Whether producing a unique item or manufacturing quantities of product, the process of going from sheep to shawl offers unlimited opportunities for developing skills of all sorts.

> Weaving and cloth construction require perceptual skills, dexterity, and coordination to a greater or lesser extent, depending on the method. They also require cognitive skills to follow pattern directions. Some materials can cause skin irritations.

Yarn Making

You will need:

Wool fleece
Cards (wire brushes)
Drop spindle or spinning wheel

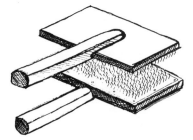

Carding

Carding aligns the fibers and removes seeds, burrs, and soil from natural wool or fleece.

1. Hold two cards opposite one another. Place a handful of fleece on one card; pull the cards against one another in opposite directions to draw the fibers out so they are parallel to one another.

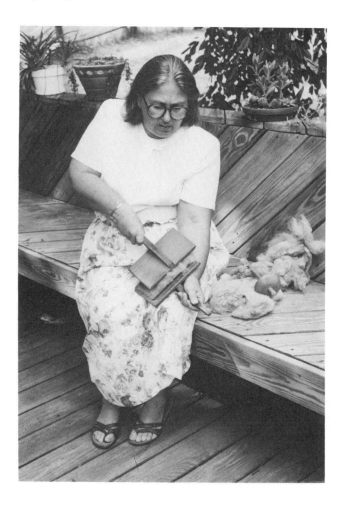

2. Remove the fleece by reversing one card and brushing the fibers in the opposite direction.

3. Repeat the process numerous times until the wool is clean of seeds and dirt and the fibers are aligned.

4. Carefully remove the fleece from the cards forming a roll, or rulag.

Commercial rulag is available for those who prefer to skip this process and get right to spinning. Quilt batting also may be used as an alternative.

> This activity requires considerable bilateral strength and coordination.

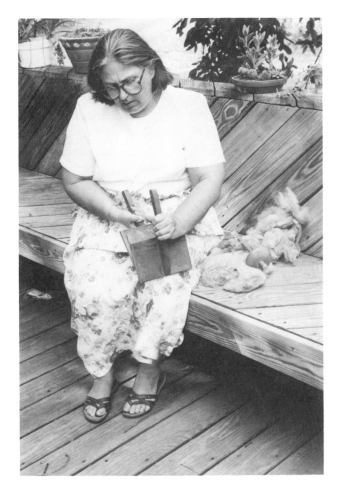

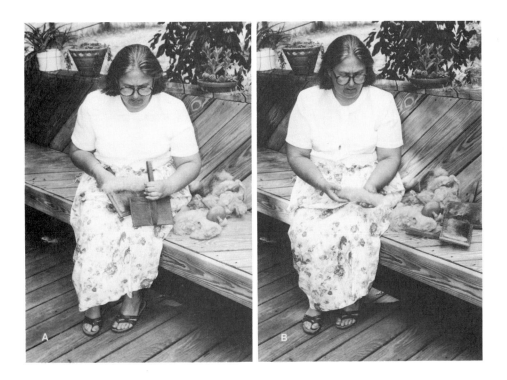

Spinning

Spinning is a technique used to intertwine fibers, strengthening them so they can be used to produce cloth. The simplest method is to attach a weight such as a rock to the fibers and set it spinning. As the weight spins, the fibers wrap around each other forming thread. Gravity and inertia are used to create the yarn.

A simple adaptation of this gravity-operated tool is called a drop spindle. Drop spindles are included among the artifacts of many ancient peoples. They were made of various materials, such as wood or ceramic. They are still commercially available today and are usually made of finely finished wood. Drop spindles are designed so they can be spun rapidly, twisting the fibers. The yarn can be wrapped onto the spindle's stem, enabling yardage to be produced.

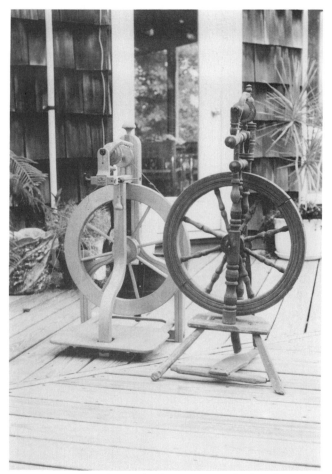

Figure 6–25. Modern Schacht spinning wheel and antique Austrian castle wheel.

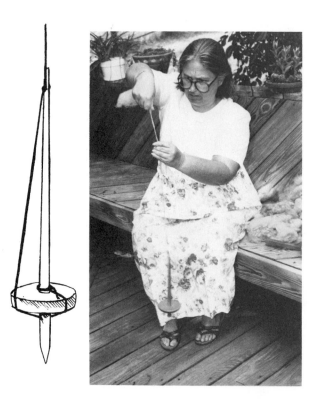

The spinning wheel is a further improvement on the drop spindle. Most wheels are operated by a foot treadle, leaving the hands free to spin. Tension controls on the wheel allow the spinner to vary yarn production in numerous ways. Yarn also can be plied, that is, the threads spun together in multiples of two or three. Plying yarn increases both its strength and the number of design possibilities.

Antique and modern spinning wheels come in a number of different styles, many of which are very beautifully crafted (Fig. 6–25). Spinning remains a popular craft in many places, particularly in rural communities where fleece is readily available. Some modern spinners use electrified spinning wheels.

Using a spinning wheel requires the coordination of upper and lower extremities. Once one becomes proficient at spinning, it is a very relaxing activity because of the repetitive rocking motion provided by the treadling.

Skeining

Spun yarn is skeined to keep it from tangling. A number of interesting tools have been designed for making skeins, but yarn can simply be wound around a chair back. Tie the skeins in several places to keep them from coming undone. Once a skein is tied, it can be washed and dyed. Later, skeins are wound into balls.

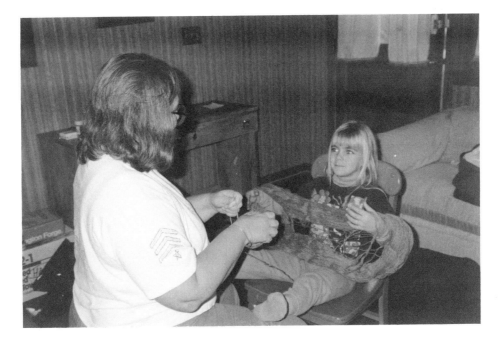

Washing

Wash wool carefully with mild soap, and rinse it well. Do not squeeze the yarn or handle it excessively. Slowly raise and lower the temperature of the bath, because sudden changes in temperature and excess handling cause wool to become hard and inflexible. In fact, felt is made by pouring hot water through fleece and pounding the fleece until it forms a solid mass.

Dyeing

Some people enjoy preparing dyes from materials collected in nature. Simply using tea or onion skins provides a dye bath of a beautiful golden color. Dandelion heads, acorns, goldenrod, and berries also will produce lovely colors. However, natural dye baths require mordants, or fixatives, in addition to the coloring agents. Varying mordants will vary the colors you get from the same natural materials. It is important to use tried and true recipes and follow them exactly, or your efforts will be apt to wash out.

More permanent and richer colors can be obtained from commercial dyes than from vegetable dyes. Instructions for the use of dyes can be obtained from manufacturers, but most dyers experiment and keep recipes.

Hand-dyed yarn has great variability in color, so one should dye a sufficient amount in one dye bath for an entire single project. However, because the beauty of creating objects from hand-dyed yarn is often the variability in the colors, many weavers combine colors from different dyeings.

You will need:

2- to 3-gallon enamel dishpans
Stirrers
Glass bowls and measuring cups, pints, and quarts
Measuring spoons
Glass funnels
Rubber gloves

Prepare in a well-ventilated space as some chemicals used in dyeing are toxic.

PROCEDURES FOR DYEING

1. **Scouring**. Immerse fibers in hot, soapy water and simmer from 30 to 45 minutes. Cool and rinse in warm water.

2. **Mordanting**. Mordants are metallic salts. They are used in combination with dyes to make colors permanent. Tin produces bright colors; copperas (iron or ferrous sulfate) darkens and is used for green, purple, and black; chrome (potassium dichromate) is used for blue, gold, and rusts; blue vitriol (copper sulfate) is used for greenish tones.

Mordanting can be done before, during, or after dyeing. Dissolve mordant into liquid. Add yarns and simmer 30 minutes from 180° to 210°. Cool the yarns in the liquid. Rinse in warm water until the rinse is clear. Then drain and hang in the shade to dry. Or, combine mordant, dye, and yarn and follow procedure below.

The basic dye recipe follows:

1 lb yarn
Mordant*
Natural ingredients*
4 Tbs. tartaric acid
½ c. Glauber's salt

Boil fruit or other natural ingredients in several gallons of water. Strain out the solids. Add wet, mordanted wool to the liquid, or add mordant to dye bath and undyed wool. Simmer 30 minutes. Add tartaric acid and Glauber's salts. Simmer 30 minutes more. Cool in dye bath, rinse until clear. Hang in the shade to dry.

Using Kool-aid is a simple method of dyeing yarn into beautiful colors. Wet the yarn; put it into a roaster pan in the oven at 200°F for approximately 1 to 2 hours. Allow to cool, remove yarn from dye bath, rinse in tepid water until clear, and hang to dry.

Commercial Yarns

Beautiful yarns of every description are commercially available and are commonly used for most yarncrafts. Yarns come in different weights, textures, and colors. When following a pattern, be sure to purchase the correct weight yarn; otherwise, your gauge, and therefore the size of the item you are making, will be incorrect. Be sure to purchase enough yarn of the same dye lot to complete your project so that the color is identical throughout.

Yarncraft Techniques

Many yarncrafts are used to create fabrics of various sorts. All are built on the same idea of twisting or looping

Table 6-3. NATURAL INGREDIENTS AND MORDANTS

Red—pokeweed berries and alum mordant
Pink—red, ripe, ornamental crab apples and alum mordant
Yellow—chrysanthemums, marigolds, zinnias, yellow or red onion skins and tin mordant
Blues—elderberries and chrome mordant
Green—floribunda rose and copperas mordant
Olive—goldenrod and copperas mordant
Lavender—blackberries and alum mordant
Purple—elderberries and tin mordant
Tan—coffee grounds and alum mordant

---

*See Table 6-3.

yarn together so that it will not unravel and so that it can be used to create cloth for many purposes. A selection of commonly used yarncraft techniques are described below.

Latch Hooking

Latch, or latchet, hooking, also known as rya, is of Scandinavian origin, although a similar method is used to produce rugs in the Orient. Latch hooking produces a pile fabric similar to that used for making carpeting. Short cuts of yarn are individually knotted onto a canvas underlayment to produce a fabric of depth and dimension. People use latch hooking to produce attractive pillows, wall hangings, and area rugs. Latch hooking is readily portable and lends itself to the easy production of beautiful designs.

You will need:

Canvas
Cut yarn or yarn cutter
Masking tape
Latchet hook

1. Cut a piece of canvas 2 inches wider than the desired finished size of your project.
2. Tape the edges of the canvas to keep it from unravelling.
3. Create a design for your project on graph paper, or simply draw a geometric design directly onto the canvas with indelible inks so it will not bleed when washed.
4. Mark the top of your project with a thread. Always keep this edge up so the pile retains the same direction throughout.
5. Begin working 1 inch from the border, leaving the remaining edge for finishing with a hem. Leave 1 inch from each edge for finishing.
6. Obtain cut yarn from commercial sources or cut the yarn to length from worsted weight yarn. If you are cutting your own yarn, wrap it around a piece of cardboard and cut it with scissors to be sure all the lengths are the same, or use a special tool designed for this purpose.
7. Insert the latchet hook under a horizontal thread and up to the face of the canvas.
8. Wrap one strand of yarn under the latchet hook handle. Hold each end and bring them up to the hook.
9. Draw both ends of the yarn through the hook. Pull the ends back through the canvas, slipping them through the loop. Pull taut.
10. Repeat in each hole across the row.
11. Continue in each row until finished, changing yarn colors according to the design as you work.

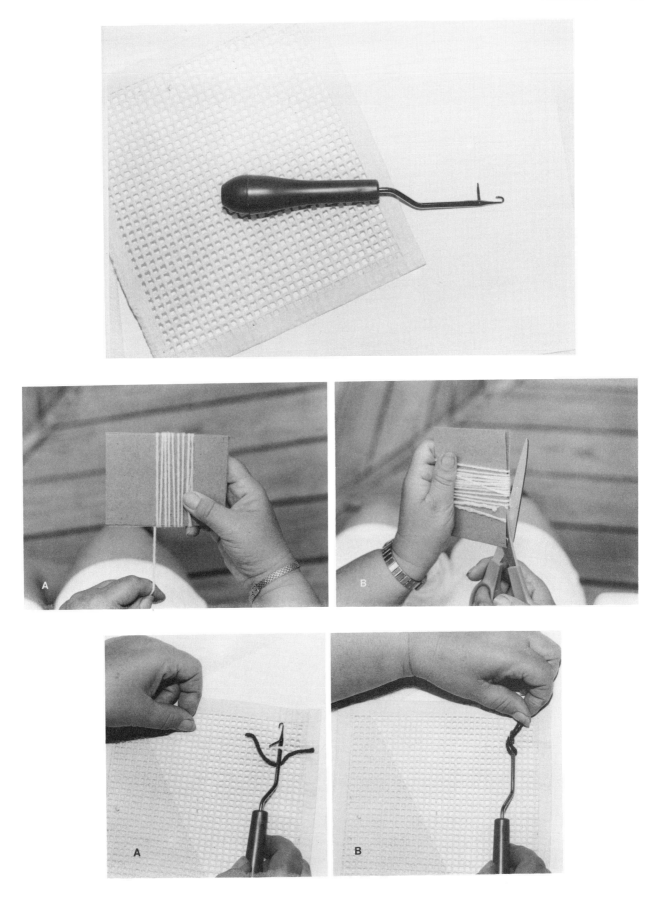

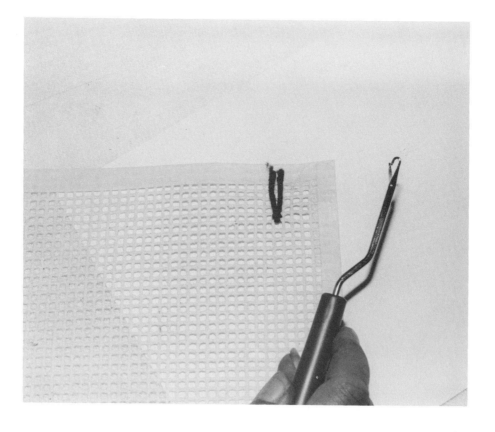

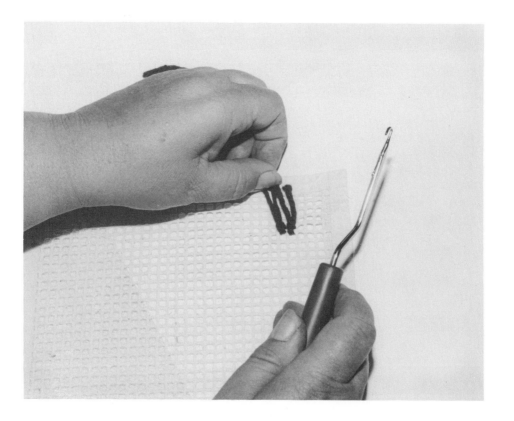

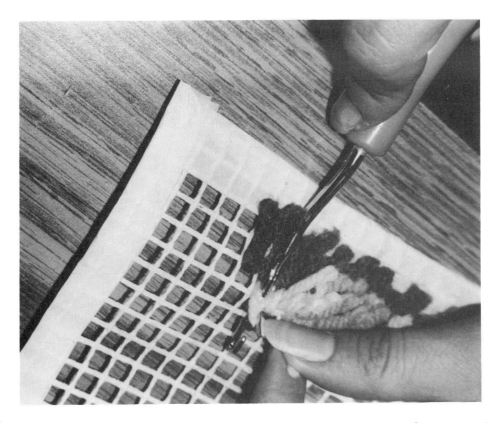

Macramé

Macramé, also known as cord knotting, is a craft that dates back to the earliest peoples who used it for creating nets for fishing. It reached its zenith among the sailors of history. Skillful handling of rope was a vital part of the sailor's work day. On long sea voyages, sailors turned their skill with rope toward more leisurely pursuits.

Macramé remains a popular activity. Attractive items for the home such as curtains, lampshades, plant hangers, and belts can be made from macramé (Fig. 6–26). The author owns a magnificent "chupah," or wedding canopy, made of macramé (Fig. 6–27).

Net bags, commonly used in Europe for shopping, are gaining popularity in this country with the increasing awareness of the need for protecting the environment.

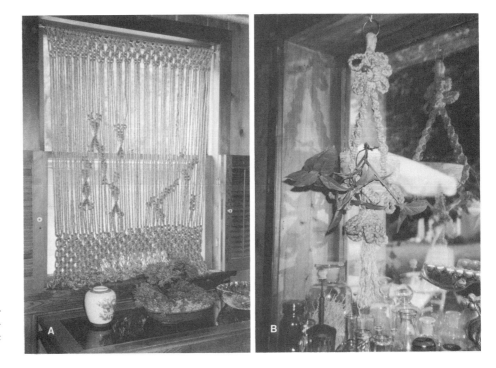

Figure 6–26. (*A*) Macramé window curtains, by author. (*B*) Macramé plant holder, by Suzanne Leichtling.

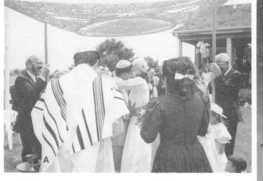

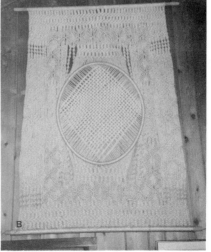

Figure 6–27. Wedding canopy (chupah), by Suzanne Leichtling.

Cord knotting requires bilateral strength, dexterity, and perceptual proficiency. Some materials are dusty and can cause respiratory distress, and others are rough on the hands. Masks and gloves can be used to avoid these irritations. Check hands carefully for signs of redness. Also, be aware that cording material can be dangerous in the hands of suicidal or homicidal patients who could injure themselves or others.

PLANT HANGER

You will need:

6 pieces of jute, each 7 feet long
Brass ring (2 inches)

Special terminology:

Lark's head
Half-knots—left over right *or* right over left.
Square knots—left over right *and* right over left.
Sinnet—series of knots.

1. Fold one 7-foot length of cord into 2 equal halves.
2. Insert the fold of the cord into a brass ring.
3. Draw the ends of the cord through the loop and pull until taut. This is called a lark's head.
4. Repeat with another 7-foot length of cord, creating 4 working cords. Make certain all loops are drawn through in the same direction, or alternate for special effect.
5. Attach the ring to a hook or post because you will need both hands to work (Fig. 6–28). Tie the middle

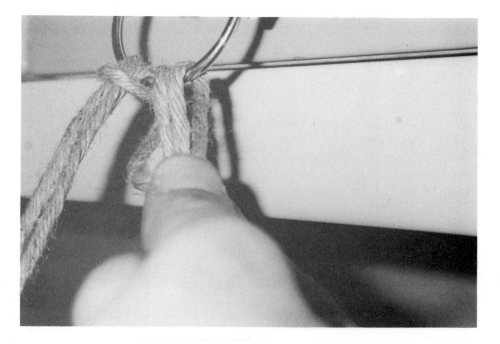

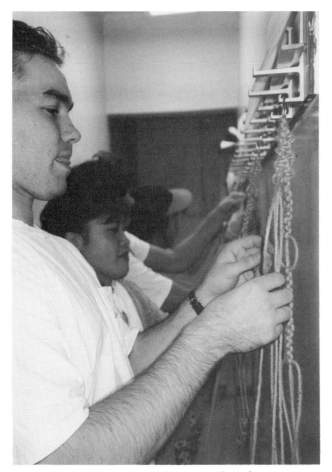

Figure 6–28. Occupational therapy students learning macramé.

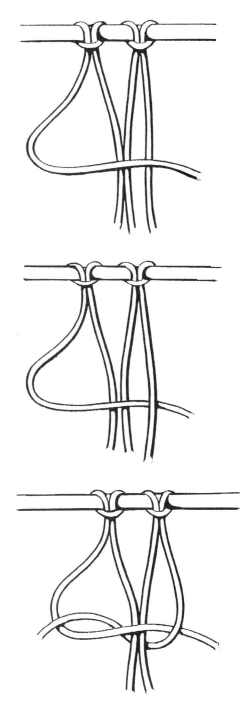

two cord ends to a belt around your waist to keep the core cords taut.

6. Working with the 2 outer cords, tie 3½ inches of half-knots as follows: Cross the left cord over 2 middle-core cords so they resemble the number "4." Cross the right cord over the left cord, under the core cords, and come up through the loop made by the left cord. Pull both ends tight.

7. Continue making these half-knots to produce a twisted sinnet 3½ inches long.

8. Now make 3½ inches of square knots. Two half-knots, one in each direction (4 and ꝭ), form a square knot. Starting with the right cord, make a half-knot. This time the figure 4 will be reversed (ꝭ). Then make a half-knot on the left side. Continue alternating knots for 3½ inches.

9. When you have worked 3½ inches of square knots, make the next square knot 2 inches below the others.

10. Push the knot up on the core cords to make a loop that protrudes on either side.

11. Continue working in square knots until the work measures 6 inches.

12. Add two additional cords to the ring with lark's heads.

13. Repeat the process from the beginning.

14. Repeat with a third group of cords.

15. You now have 12 cords. Take cords 3, 4, 5, and 6, and make a square knot 3 inches below.

16. Repeat this process using cords 7, 8, 9, and 10.

17. Repeat again using cords 11, 12, 1, and 2. At this point, all cords will be joined to make a circle.

18. Move 3 inches down on the cord and starting with any two sets, make a square knot using those 2 cords from each set which are closest to each other. Repeat in this fashion until 3 knots are tied.

19. Move 4½ inches down and tie all cords together. Leave a tail of 7 inches, and trim.

Knitting

TIMES AND EVENTS. Knitting is a traditional yarncraft in many places in the world. It achieved its greatest fame in the cold climates of northern Europe, particularly in Scandinavia and the British Isles, although its origins are attributed to the eastern Mediterranean lands. It is thought that wandering nomads sat astride their camels and knitted fabrics while crossing the desert as early as 1000 B.C.E. Knitting is primarily used to produce articles of clothing such as sweaters, scarves, and hats. It lends itself to creative design both in stitchery and color.

Knitting is extremely portable, needing only two needles to create many different objects. While traditional knitting is ordinarily done with needles pointed at one end and capped at the other, several double-pointed needles or one circular needle can be used.

Knitting is done one stitch at a time. All knitting is composed of two stitches, knit and purl. Every knitting pattern is simply a combination of these two stitches. Once basic knitting skills are learned, they can be used to create a wide variety of objects.

Knitting can also be done with a knitting machine, row by row. While knitting machines can be hand operated, industry adapted them to be driven by electricity. Productivity in the knitting industry has been greatly enhanced by computerization, enabling high levels of automaticity in manufacturing.

While knitting can be used to create all kinds of clothing and other objects, the directions shown here are limited to the production of a hand-knitted sampler using two needles, the most common type of knitting. Some beginners may prefer to start out making a scarf, so their first project is one they can wear. An attractive scarf can be made of ombré, a multicolored yarn, using one stitch throughout.

Knitting can be worked "right-handed" or "left-handed." These directions are given right-handed, as is customary. However, because knitting is a bilateral task, there is little difference; both hands are used with dexterity. Yarn can be held in a number of ways. Knitters generally have their own preferred style of working. Hold the yarn the way you find most comfortable.

Knitting is a bilateral task. However, it can be adapted as a unilateral activity by using a vise to hold one of the needles.

Therapists should be able to adapt themselves to the needs and customs of their patients. Once they become experienced knitters, they should familiarize themselves with different styles of working. Some knitters find that they become less tired if they switch from one style of knitting to another from time to time.

Because many older persons can knit and many younger ones cannot, learning to knit from older patients is a very therapeutic experience for the teacher-patient.

You will need:

Yarn
Knitting needles
Tapestry needle
Measuring tape

Abbreviations:

Knit	K
Purl	P
Increase	Inc
Decrease	Dec
Repeat	*

CASTING ON. There are a number of ways to cast on stitches. This is one simple way for a beginner to learn.

1. Hold 2 needles together in the right hand, casting the stitches onto both needles at once.

2. Hold the yarn in the left hand, looped over the forefinger and thumb.

3. Insert the needles below the thumb yarn and over the yarn that runs behind the forefinger.

4. Draw the farther yarn back under the thumb yarn.

5. Release the yarn from the finger and thumb.

6. Pull the stitch taut around the needles.

7. Continue casting on until there are 40 stitches on the needle.

8. Slip one needle out, leaving all 40 stitches on the remaining needle. The stitches will slip easily back and forth along the needle, making it easy to begin to knit.

KNIT

1. Hold the needle with the stitches on it in your left hand. Hold the empty needle in your right hand.

2. *Keeping the yarn behind the work, insert the right needle through the first stitch from its left to its right.

3. Wrap the yarn around the point of the right needle.

4. Draw the yarn through the stitch forming a new stitch.

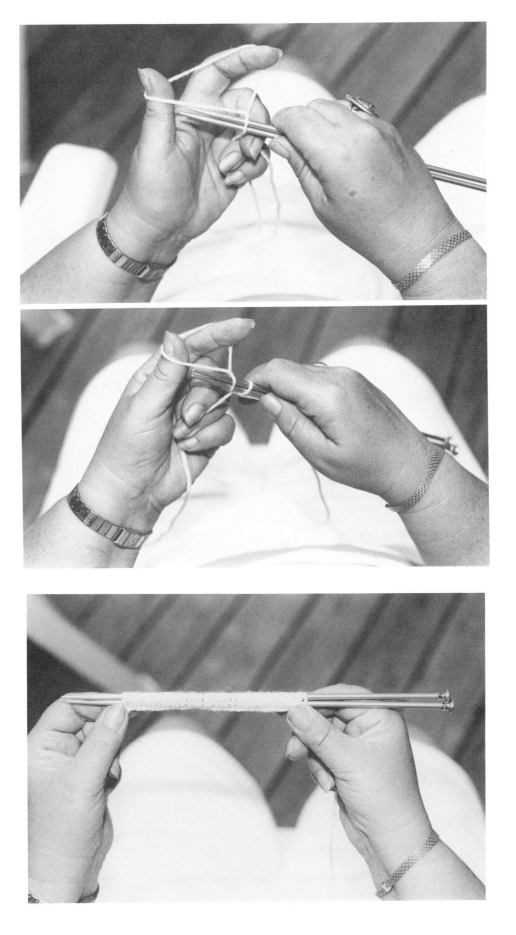

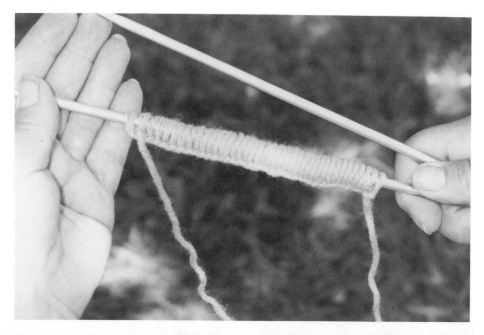

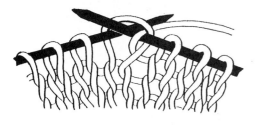

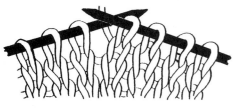

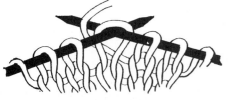

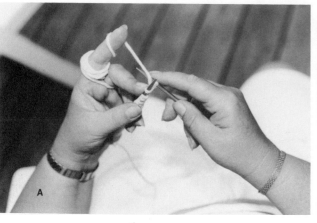

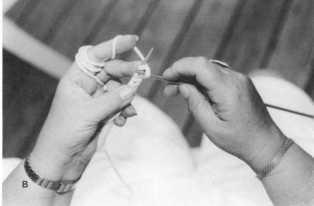

5. Slip the old stitch off the left needle. Repeat from * across the row until all stitches are on the right-hand needle.

6. To begin a new row, switch needles into the opposite hands and continue from * across the row.

When a project is made of knitting alone, the stitch is called a garter stitch. Both sides of the work are horizontally ribbed and identical in appearance.

PURL

1. Hold the needles and yarn as you did when knitting, but keep the yarn in front of the work.

2. *Insert the right needle into the first stitch from right to left, passing the right needle in front of the left needle.

3. Drop the yarn over the right needle and draw the yarn back through the stitch forming a new stitch.

4. Slip the old stitch off the left needle.

5. Continue from * across the row until all the stitches are on the right-hand needle.

6. To begin a new row, switch each needle into the opposite hand.

When working purl alone. the work will appear identical to the garter stitch; however, the garter stitch is ordinarily done using knit alone.

STOCKINETTE. Alternate 1 row of knit and 1 row of purl. Stockinette stitch has a right and a wrong side. The right side is smooth, the wrong side is pebbled, similar in appearance to a garter stitch. Stockinette is the most commonly used stitch. With few exceptions, the knit or smooth side is the side used for the outside of the garment.

RIBBING. Ribbing is used when elasticity is desired, such as for neck trim, cuffs, and waistbands. Alternate 2 knit stitches and 2 purl stitches in each row. This pattern can be varied according to the design of the item being made, by changing the number of stitches in the rib.

INCREASING. To shape a garment it is necessary to vary the number of stitches on a row. To increase, begin as you would to knit, but do not drop the stitch off the left needle. Instead, treat the remaining part of the stitch as if it were a separate stitch. That is, enter the back of the stitch and knit it again.

You will have made 2 stitches from 1 stitch. One can increase at any point along the row, depending on the pattern.

DECREASING. To decrease, knit 2 stitches together as if they were one. Decreasing can be done at the beginning or end of the row, or any point along the row, according to the pattern.

BINDING OFF

1. Knit the 1st and 2nd stitches.

2. Pass the 1st stitch on the right needle over the 2nd stitch, and drop it off.

3. Knit the next stitch off the left needle onto the right.

4. Pass the 1st stitch over the 2nd stitch on the right needle.

5. Continue binding off according to the directions, or until the row is complete.

6. Cut the yarn, leaving about 3 inches. Draw the end through the remaining stitch. Pull taut. Tuck in all loose threads.

SAMPLER

1. Cast on 40 stitches.

2. Work 10 rows of knit.

3. Work 10 rows of purl.

4. Stockinette 10 rows.

5. Do 10 rows of ribbing.

6. Knit squares as follows: Row 1—* K5, P5 repeat across the row. Row 2—P5, K5 repeat across the row**. Repeat from * to ** 3 more times, ending at row 8. Row 9—***P5, K5 repeat across the row. Row 10—K5, P5 across the row. Repeat from *** 3 more times.

7. Bind off.

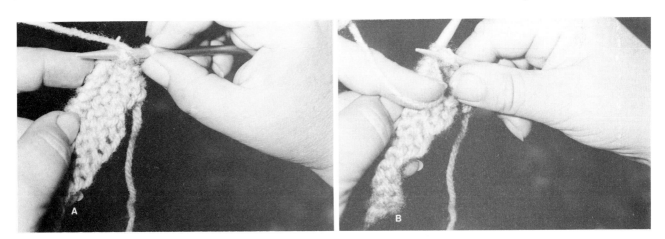

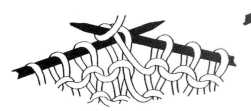
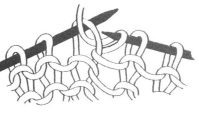
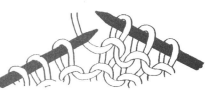

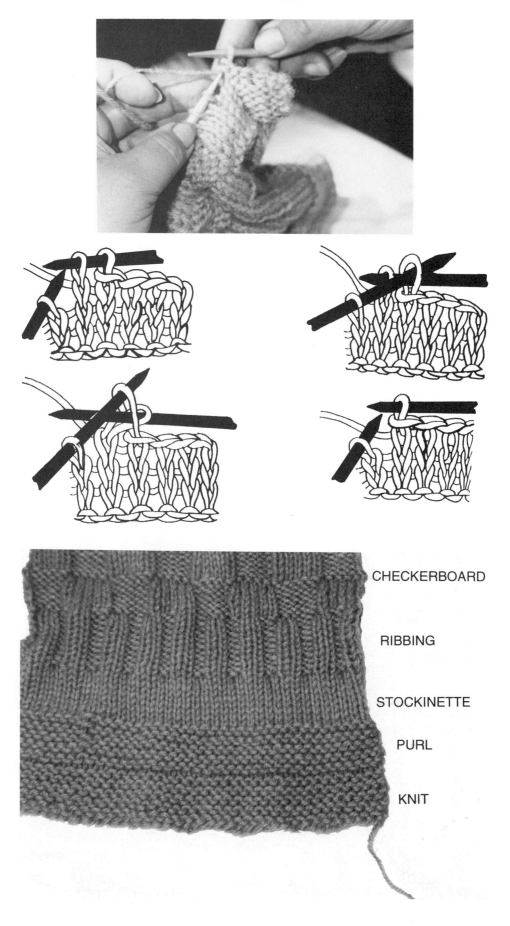

CHECKERBOARD

RIBBING

STOCKINETTE

PURL

KNIT

GAUGE. Each knitter knits at a different tension. Because some knitters knit more tightly than others and each yarn is somewhat thicker or thinner, it is necessary to determine the gauge before casting on. Knit a small square of the yarn you will be using. Measure the knitting to determine the number of lines and stitches per inch. Experienced knitters sometimes forego the use of a ruler and use their thumb as a measuring tool. Measure your thumb to determine exactly how long an inch is.

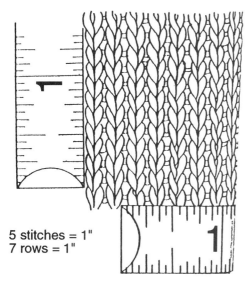

5 stitches = 1"
7 rows = 1"

SCARF

1. Cast on 40 stitches of worsted weight, 4-ply, or Germantown, yarn.
2. Knit until the scarf is the length you want.
3. Bind off.
4. Fringe as follows.

FRINGE

1. Cut a piece of cardboard 4 × 6 inches or use a book.
2. Wind yarn 6 times around the 6-inch dimension.
3. Cut the yarn on one side leaving 6 strands 12 inches in length.
4. Fold the threads in half. Insert a crochet hook into the end of the scarf at the corner.
5. Pull the fringe partially through the scarf at the center of the threads forming a loop.
6. Insert the ends of the fringe through the loop. Pull snug.
7. Continue adding fringes, spacing them evenly across the row.
8. Fringe the other end of the scarf.

Hand-knitted objects are highly valued. Once you know these basic techniques, you can begin to make garments of all sorts, from socks to suits. Patterns are commercially available in knitting shops and must be followed precisely. Hold off on designing your own patterns until you become expert.

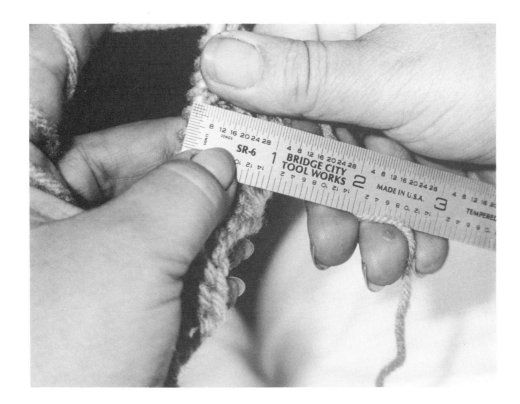

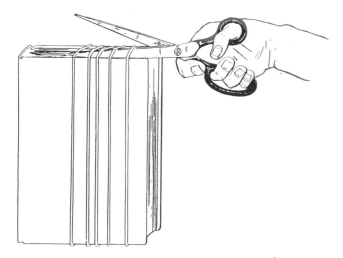

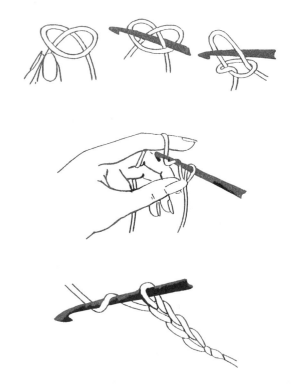

Crocheting

Crocheting is similar to knitting, but it is done with one needle—a crochet hook. Crocheting is commonly used to make garments and blankets called afghans. There are many elaborate stitches made by looping the yarn around itself. Very beautiful items can be made from this simple process (Fig. 6–29).

ABBREVIATIONS

Chain	ch
Single crochet	sc
Half-double crochet	hdc
Double crochet	dc
Loop	lp
Yarn over	yo

CHAINING. Start by making a slip knot on the crochet hook about 6 inches from the end of the yarn. Pull tight. Hold the hook between the right index finger and thumb. Wrap the yarn around the left ring or index finger to hold it taut. Catch the yarn with the hook and pull it through the lp. Repeat, making the ch as long as is called for in the pattern.

SINGLE CROCHET. Insert the hook into the second ch from the hook, under both strands of yarn. Draw up a lp. Draw the yarn over the hook and pull through the 2 lps, completing the sc. Skipping a stitch, insert hook into the next stitch and repeat according to the pattern.

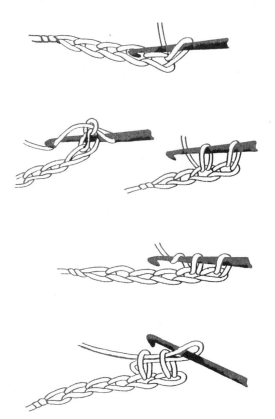

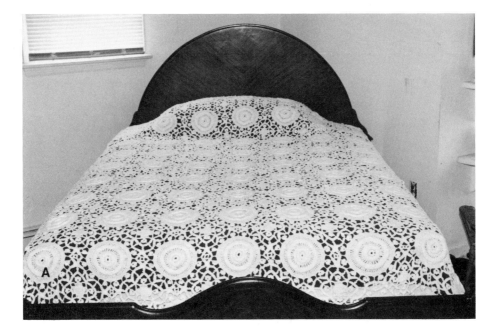

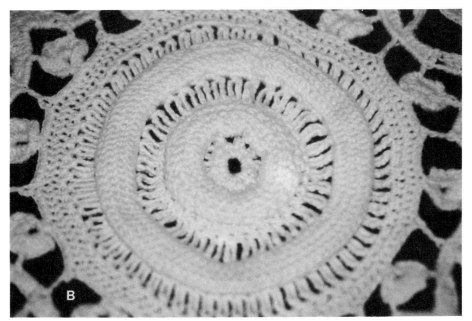

Figure 6–29. Crocheted bedspread and detail, by Sylvia Borgman.

HALF-DOUBLE CROCHET. With yarn over hook, insert hook into 3rd ch. Draw up a lp. Draw yarn over hook. Pull through the 3 lps, completing the hdc. Repeat according to the pattern.

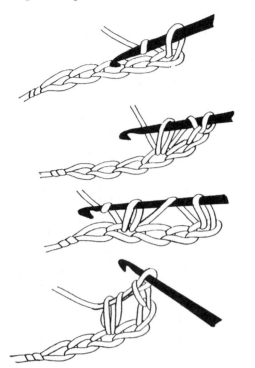

DOUBLE CROCHET. With yarn over hook, insert hook into 4th ch. Draw up a lp. Wrap yarn over hook. Draw yarn through 2 lps. Yo again and through the last 2 lps on the hook, completing the dc.

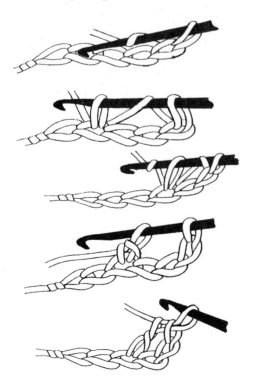

Weaving

Weaving is a technique of interlacing vertical and horizontal threads. The vertical threads are the warp, and the horizontal threads are called the weft, woof, or filler. Many techniques of weaving have been designed using the same underlying concepts, producing fabric for many uses.

TERMINOLOGY

Warp. Vertical threads.

Weft, woof, filler. Horizontal threads.

Warping board. Wooden frame into which dowel rods are set. Used to measure warp.

Heddles. Moveable "needles" that hold and guide each warp thread.

Heddle eye. The hole through which the thread runs.

Sley hook. Tool used to thread warp through heddles and reed.

Warp beam. Front beam of the loom.

Weft or cloth beam. Back beam of the loom.

Ratchets. Mechanism used to tighten warp on the loom.

Levers. Mechanism used to change sheds on a table loom.

Treadles. Mechanism used to change sheds on a floor loom.

Reed. Measured frame governing the width of fabric.

Dent. Spaces in the reed through which warp runs.

Beam. Front and back structures of loom.

Shuttle. Tool used to pass weft through the warp.

Boat shuttle. Specialized shuttle resembling a small boat.

Selvedge. Edges of fabric formed as weaving progresses.

Harness or frame. Moveable wooden structure into which heddles sit. Can be raised or lowered to form a shed.

Shed. An opening formed between groups of threads when the harness is raised or lowered, through which the weft is thrown.

FRAME WEAVING. Weaving frames are made of different kinds of materials. Cardboard can be used for small projects. A wooden frame can be used for larger projects. Wooden stretchers are available at art supply stores, come in graduated lengths, and can give you exactly the size frame you need.

Cardboard Weaving Frame. Simple cardboard weaving frames are commercially available but can be easily made. Score a piece of strong cardboard with slits ¼ inch apart top and bottom. This card is now a small weaving loom. Thread the loom with warp thread.

1. Insert the thread into the first slit from back to front, wrapping the end to keep it from slipping out.

2. Draw the thread down along the face of the card, securing the thread in the slit directly below.

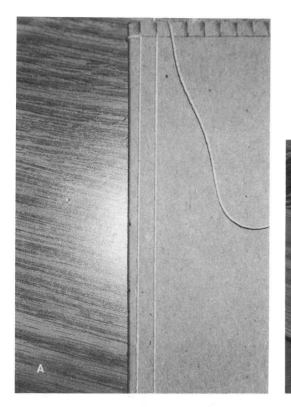

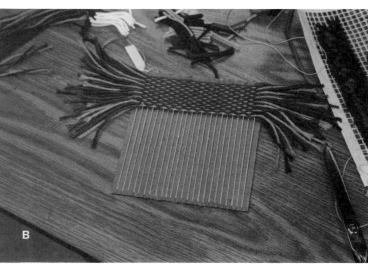

3. Pass the thread behind the cardboard, coming forward into the adjacent slit.

4. Run the thread up to the top, inserting it into the second slit.

5. Continue threading the loom in this manner so the warp threads run parallel up and down the face of the entire card. No warp thread should run along the back of the card.

6. Secure the thread at the last corner.

Wooden Frame Weaving

1. Mark the top and bottom edges of the frame at regular intervals (e.g., every ¼ inch), being sure the top and bottom marks are aligned evenly.

2. Notch the frame where it is marked with a pen knife or file, or nail small brads into the frame.

3. Wrap the frame as described above. Several weaving methods are possible using this kind of loom.

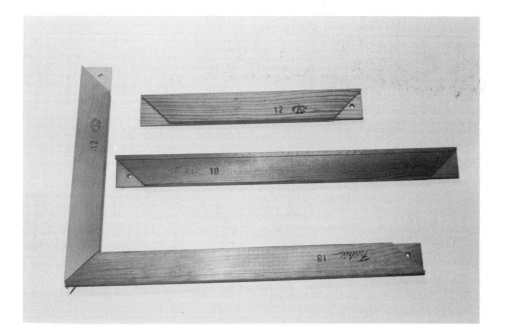

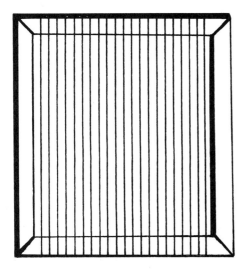

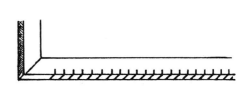

Method 1. Draw a pattern on a paper that has been cut to fit the loom. Slip it under the threads to guide your weaving, securing it to the frame with tape.

A small shuttle can be made either from a tongue depressor, by notching the ends, or from a long piece of cardboard. A long weaver's needle also can be used.

Select appropriate yarns for your design. Weave under and over each alternating thread, changing the colors of the weft according to the design. Alternate the threads when weaving the next row. When you change colors on the same line, interlock the weft threads by twisting them around each other to secure them.

Be careful not to pull your work in on the sides. Good weaving is judged by the straightness of the selvedge. To keep the edges even, lay the weft in on the diagonal.

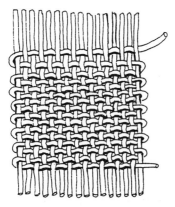

Method 2. Cut threads 4 inches longer than the width of the frame. Weave each thread through, leaving equal lengths of fringed edges on the sides. A pattern can be made by changing the colors at specified intervals.

Method 3. This method produces a pile and is used for making rugs. Designs are made by changing yarn colors as the work proceeds. Using warp cord, weave across one time, leaving the cord attached to the ball.

Cut yarn into 2½-inch lengths. Starting from the left,

place the yarn in front of the first 2 threads. Wrap the ends of the cut yarn around the outside of the warp threads, and bring the ends down through between the same threads.

Continue across the row, tying each piece of yarn over every 2 threads. At the end of each row of yarn, weave across with the warp cord. Alternate yarn rows should start with warp threads 1 and 2 or 2 and 3 to provide strength. When completed, this looks like latch hooking.

Harness Loom. The development of the moveable frame or harness loom represents a marked advance in weaving. This development enabled yard goods of unlimited designs and extensive lengths of yardage to be woven. When the harness loom was further automated by electricity, the textile industry advanced its role as a major industrial segment.

Interestingly, the French method of using punch cards that was initially devised to create elaborate Jacquard weaving designs was later adopted in the development of computers. Now, computers are used to operate looms.

The harness loom comes in table or floor varieties. While the size of the work is dictated by the size of the loom, each variety of loom operates according to the same principles. A harness loom permits one to weave myriad designs, the complexity of which can be increased as the numbers of harnesses are increased. These designs are made by treadling, or alternating, the rotation of threads. Most looms have 2 or 4 harnesses, but there can be up to 32 harnesses.

Preparing the Warp. A warping frame allows lengthy warp to be prepared in a comparatively small space. By wrapping thread back and forth on the spokes of a warping frame, the length and design of the warp can be accurately controlled. Warp is wrapped so a cross is formed by each alternating thread. Tie the warp at the cross and at several points on the warp to keep it from tangling.

Once the warp is prepared, it is ready to be threaded onto the loom.

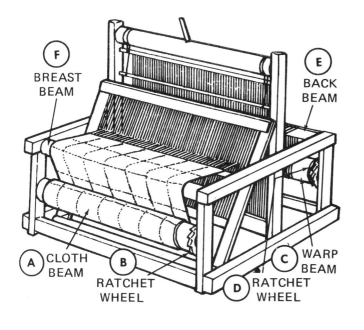

F BREAST BEAM
E BACK BEAM
A CLOTH BEAM
B RATCHET WHEEL
C WARP BEAM
D RATCHET WHEEL

Adapted from Craft Techniques in Occupational Therapy. Department of the Army, Washington, DC, 1980, pp 7-1 and 7-2.

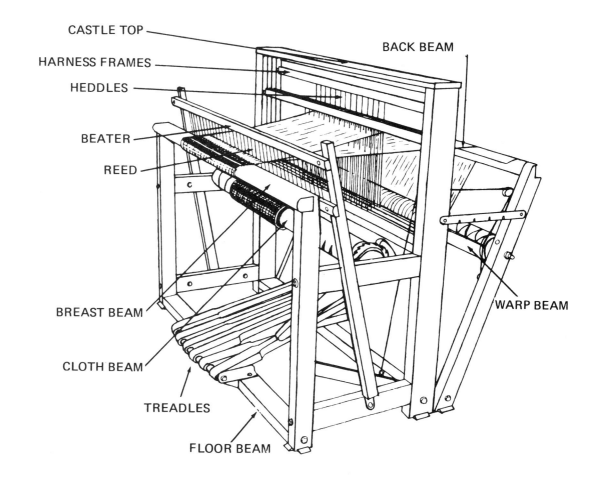

CASTLE TOP
HARNESS FRAMES
HEDDLES
BEATER
REED
BACK BEAM
WARP BEAM
BREAST BEAM
CLOTH BEAM
TREADLES
FLOOR BEAM

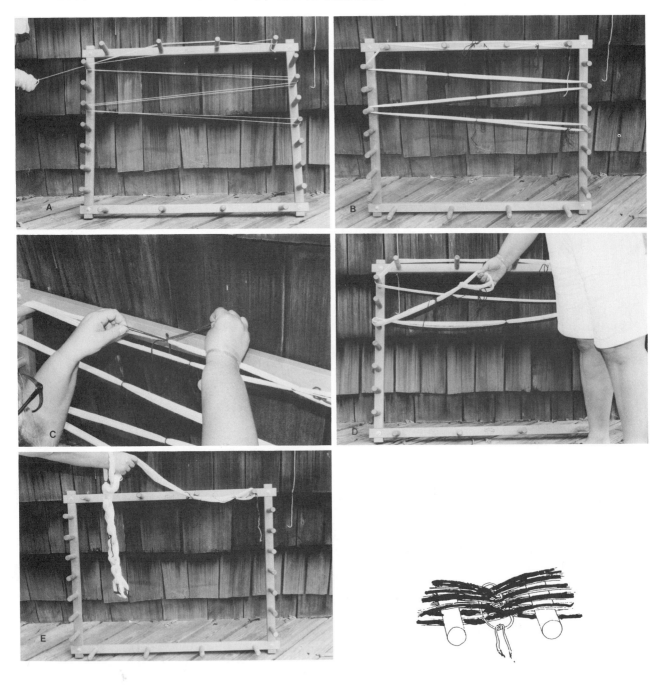

FORMULAS FOR FIGURING THE WARP

Width of project × dents per inch + selvedge = ?

Length of project + waste loom allowance, hem, or fringe = ?

Dressing the Loom. Warping a loom can be done by one person alone; however, it is done more easily and accurately by 2 people working together, one at the front and one at the back of the loom.

One reliable method for warping a 2- or 4-harness loom is as follows:

1. Lay the warp over the front beam of the loom.

2. Insert lease sticks into both sides of the cross and secure them to the sides of the loom.

3. Cut the end of the warp, creating individual threads. Note that alternating threads go under and over the lease sticks. To control the accuracy of your pattern, be careful not to cross threads over one another.

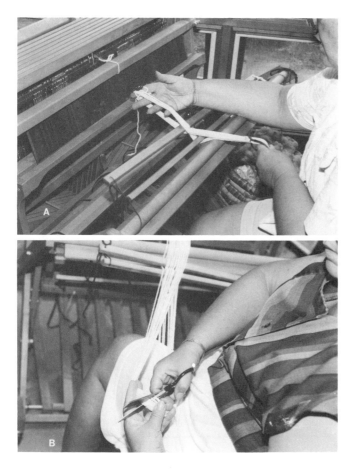

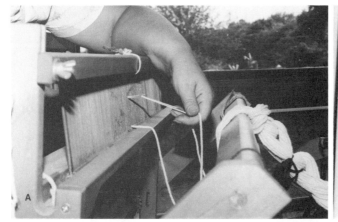

4. Start threading the warp though the reed at the center, using a sley hook. Insert the last 2 threads on each side into the same reed slot to form the selvedge.

5. Thread the heddles according to the pattern or draft. For a basic twill or tabby, on a 4-harness loom, the 1st thread goes into the front harness. The 2nd into the 2nd harness, the 3rd into the 3rd harness, the 4th into the 4th harness, the 5th into the 1st harness, and so on.

6. Tie the threads loosely in small bunches as you work to prevent them from accidentally coming loose.

7. Tie the warp onto the back beam, evenly distributing the threads across the rod.

8. You are now ready to wrap the warp. Cut brown wrapping paper (grocery bags are good for this task) to insert between the threads as you wrap, to help keep the warp tension intact.

9. Slowly wrap the warp, drawing it through the heddles, reed, and lease sticks, unchaining the warp from the front as you work. When you approach the end of the chain, leave enough length to tie onto the front rod.

10. Cut the warp ends. Tie loosely.

11. Tie the warp evenly onto the front rod, adjusting the tension at each tie until it is even.

12. Begin weaving with coarse rug yarn or rag to distribute the tension. Readjust the tension by retying sections as needed. You are now ready to weave your project.

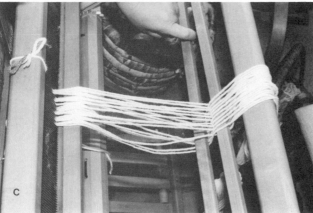

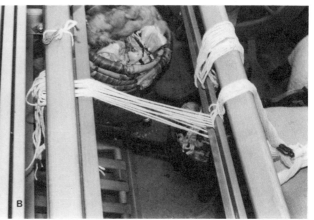

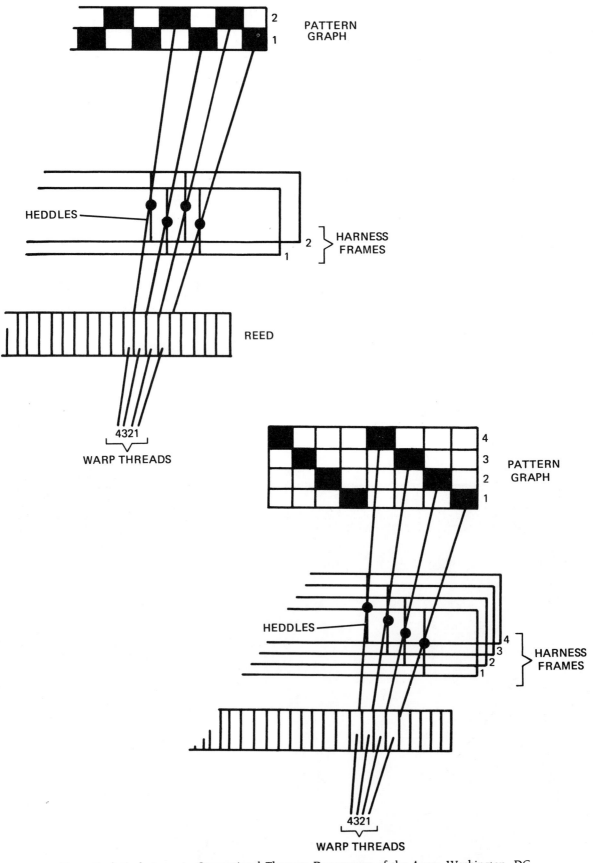

From Craft Techniques in Occupational Therapy. Department of the Army, Washington, DC, 1980, p 7-12.

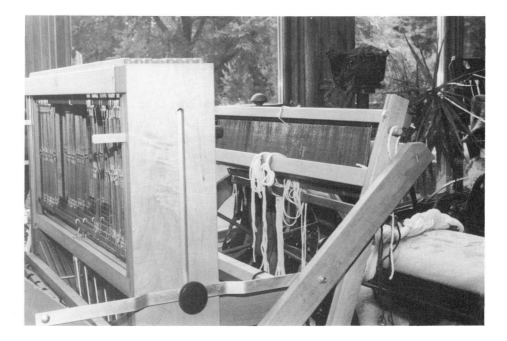

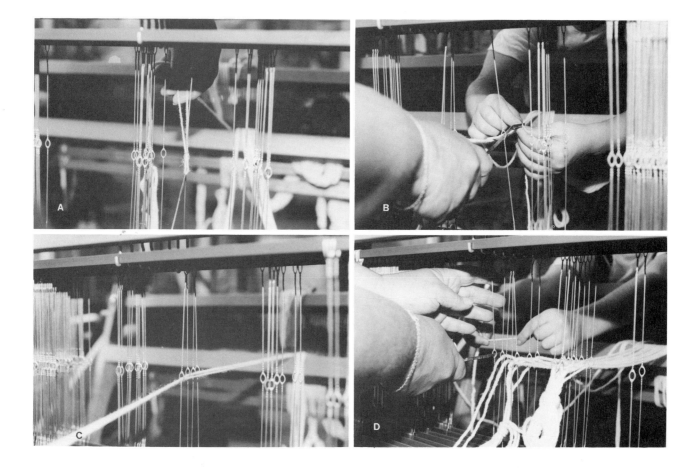

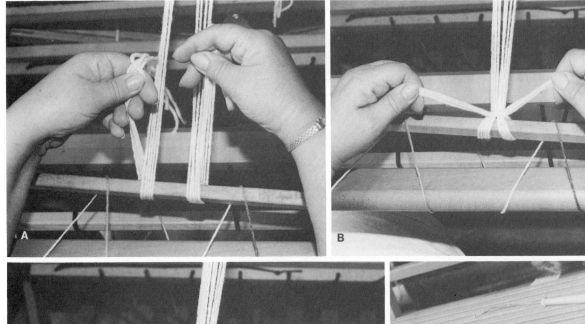

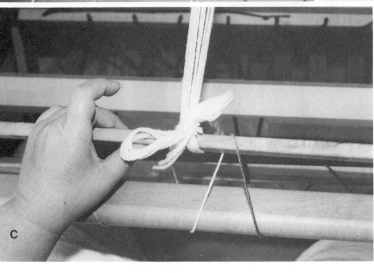

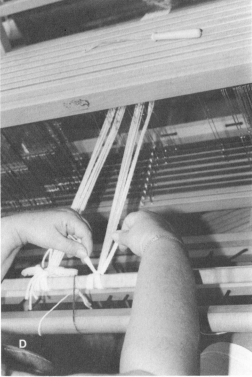

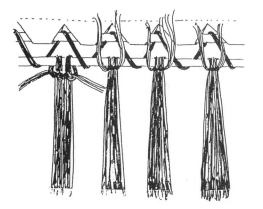

SECURING THE THREADS. To begin a thread, place the yarn through the shed, leaving a length that extends approximately 2 inches beyond the warp. Change treadles, and insert the end of the thread back through the shed for 1 inch, bringing the end up between the warp threads. Beat. Then proceed with the weaving.

When ending a thread, the same procedure is followed. Change sheds after the ending warp thread is thrown. Bring the end of the thread back through the shed and up between the warp threads approximately 1 inch in from the edge. The threads can be cut even with the weaving when the work is complete, as they have been secured by this process.

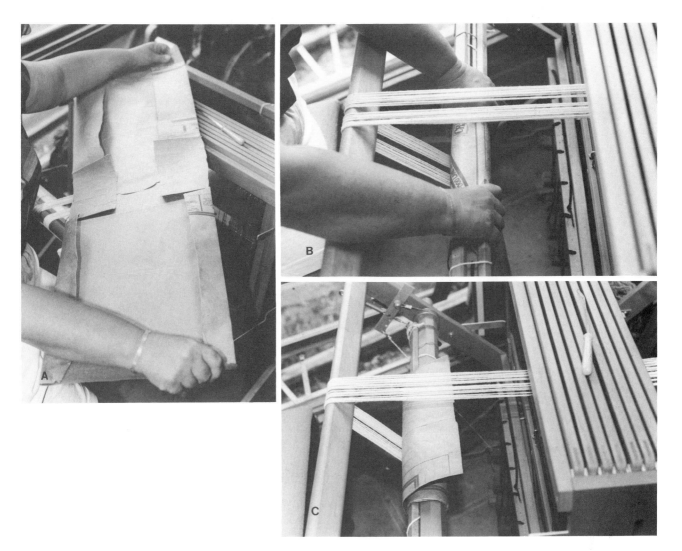

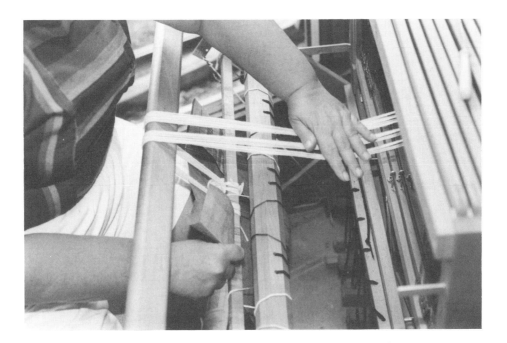

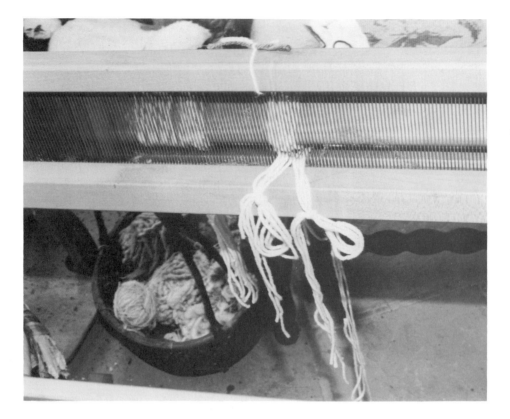

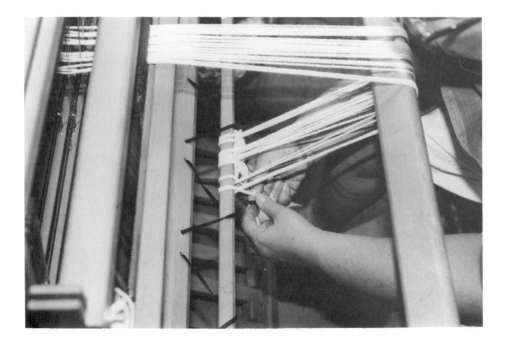

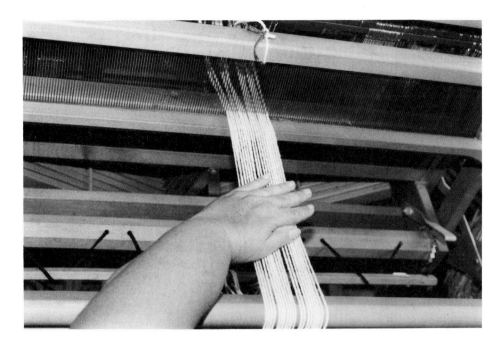

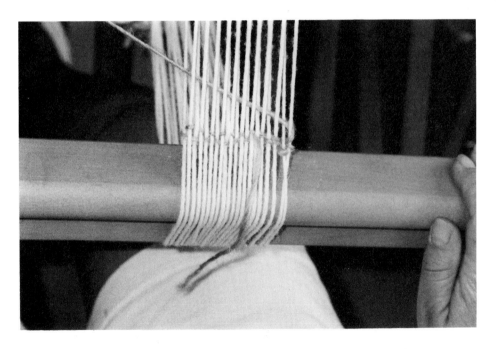

WEAVING THE PATTERN. A simple weaving pattern, called a tabby, is formed by alternately pressing harnesses 1 and 2 on a 2-harness loom. When using a 4-harness loom, press 1 and 3 together, then 2 and 4 together. When the harnesses are pressed, alternate threads raise or lower, leaving a space between the threads called a shed. The weft is thrown through this space. Many other patterns can be made by altering the treadling.

WEAVING INSTRUCTIONS

1. Press the treadles or levers.
2. Throw the shuttle through the shed.
3. Lay the weft at a diagonal to prevent the edges from pulling (see above).
4. Change sheds by pressing the alternate treadles.
5. Beat the weft with the beater.
6. Throw the shuttle, change sheds, beat. Repeat until the weaving is the length desired.

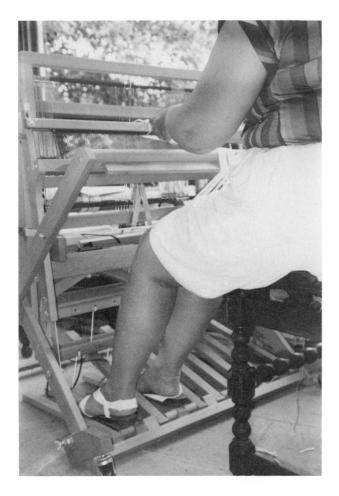

FINISHING

1. Cut the warp from the loom.
2. Thread a tapestry needle with matching yarn.
3. Stitch over the last row, picking up one warp thread in each stitch.
4. Repeat on the other end.

FRINGING

1. Divide the warp into groups of 4, 5, or 6 threads.
2. Knot each group of threads, using a needle to pull the knot snugly against the weave.
3. Lay the fringe flat on a table, marking its edge with a straightedge. Cut the fringe evenly.
4. Repeat on the reverse end.

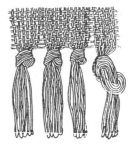

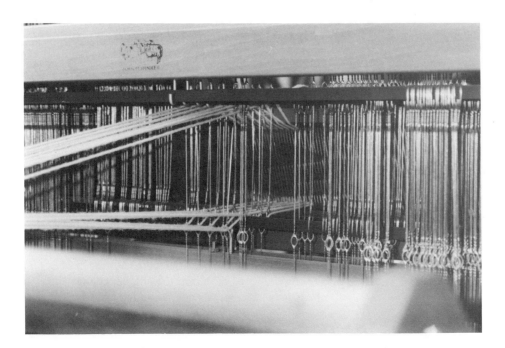

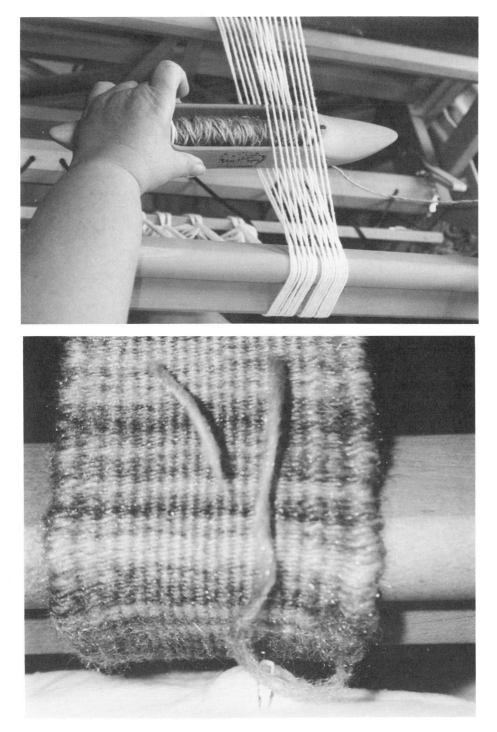

Needlework

TIMES AND EVENTS. Sewing garments is a utilitarian task that originated in ancient days when clothing was made by lacing skins together. This skill was refined, becoming the needlework used to sew fabric together.

Traditionally, women were responsible for sewing tasks within the household. Later, during the formation of towns and shops, men working as tailors assumed many of these responsibilities.

Basic needlework is a useful self-care skill for those of

Few clinics today use harness looms because of the length of time required to warp and weave projects to completion. Yet, weaving offers opportunities for creativity; decision making; building strength, endurance, coordination, and perceptual skills; and it is an excellent leisure activity. Sometimes long-term-care facilities have volunteers who come in just to warp looms. Long lengths are put on for use by multiple clients.

either gender in the modern world. While most sewing is done by machine today, skill with a needle can meet utilitarian needs, as well as provide enduring treasures.

Embroidery was an extension of the sewing arts. It was a fine art through which women expressed themselves in the years when class distinction provided wealthy women with many hours to fill with respectable tasks. The European cloisters of the Middle Ages brought needlework to a finely developed art form. Exquisite embroidery techniques of many sorts were devised, and mastery of these skills comprised a large part of the education of young women toward their role as housewives. Embroidery was used to ornament clothing and other items in the home and church. Distinctive ornamental embroidery was also done in Africa, Asia, South America, and the Scandinavian countries.

> Because self-care is a vital element of practice, learning to sew should be considered a fundamental skill. Being able to care for one's clothing is useful for everyone in modern society, regardless of gender. Buttons are always coming off!
>
> Embroidery and other fine and decorative needlecrafts are satisfying leisure crafts, requiring good vision and fine motor skills.

HAND SEWING. Fine stitching is done without making knots. Secure the thread by making 2 or 3 stitches into the same bit of fabric. Fine stitchery is evaluated by examining the back of the work as well as the front.

It is useful to assemble a sewing box that contains an assortment of items used for sewing.

You will need:

Sewing thread
Sewing needles
Straight pins
Pin cushion
Stitch ripper
Scissors
Thimble
Assorted buttons
Measuring tape

Buttons. Place the buttonhole in the closed position. Mark the spot for the button carefully with a pin. Open the garment. Sew 2 small stitches in place where the pin is. Remove the pin. In a 2-hole button, insert the needle up through one hole, down the second and back through the fabric. Repeat 3 times. Then, wrap the thread several times around the threads between the button and the fabric, forming a shank of thread. Secure the end by stitching in place several times on the reverse side of the fabric. Four-hole buttons are sewn so the visible threads lie parallel or in a cross. Whichever you select, be consistent.

Hems. Fold up the edge of the fabric ¼ inch. Press. Refold the hemmed edge to the desired length and pin it to hold it securely.

There are two ways to sew a hem. The first way is to work from right to left alternately picking up a bit of thread from top and bottom around the hem. The stitches should be barely visible on the face of the garment.

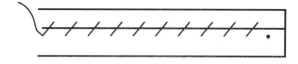

A tailor's hem is done by creating a crosshatch. Work from left to right by picking up a bit of thread from the doubled section, then the single section to the right, then the double section to the right, continuing in this way around the hem, forming a cross with each stitch. A tailor's hem tends to hold more securely.

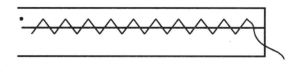

Combination Stitch. This stitch is useful in making or repairing seams. Stitch 3 small running stitches. Back stitch 1 stitch and follow with 2 more running stitches. Continue along the seam in series of 3 stitches, combining 1 back stitch and 2 running stitches. When finished, secure the thread by stitching 2 times into the same place.

Embroidery and Crewel Stitchery. These techniques are virtually identical with the exception of the materials used. Embroidery customarily is done on fine linen or cotton using floss. Crewel embroidery uses yarn on coarse fabrics.

A variety of stitches are used to create designs on the fabric. Following are a few commonly used ornamental stitches.

Ornamental Stitches

Outline

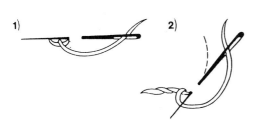

Cross-stitch

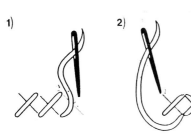

French knot

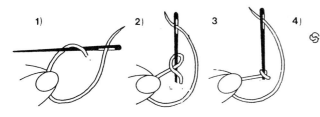

Cover stitch

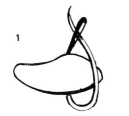

Chain or lazy daisy stitch

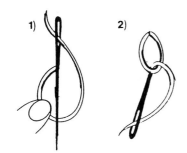

You will need:

Embroidery floss
Embroidery needles
Crewel yarn
Tapestry needles
Scissors
Embroidery hoop
Thimble
Fabric—aida cloth, embroidery, counted cross-stitch

Kits are widely available, ranging in size and complexity. Small projects are recommended for beginners. Needles and scissors can be dangerous, so a system for keeping track of them is important. Allergies to floss or crewel yarn can cause skin or respiratory problems. Embroidery hoops have been adapted to permit individuals to sew with the use of one hand only (Fig. 6–30).

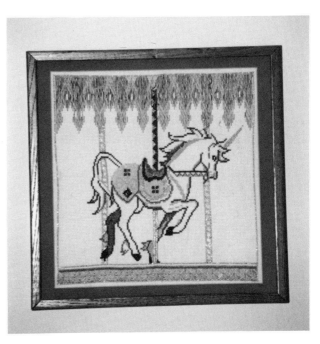

NEEDLEPOINT. Needlepoint is done by covering canvas skrim with yarn. The canvas is measured by the number of threads to the inch; the smaller the number, the coarser the skrim. Petit point and gross point are the

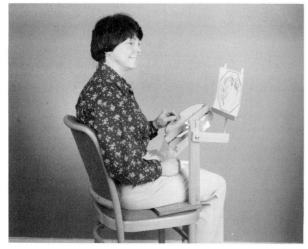

Figure 6-30. Adapted embroidery hoop. (Courtesy of S&S Worldwide, Colchester, CT.)

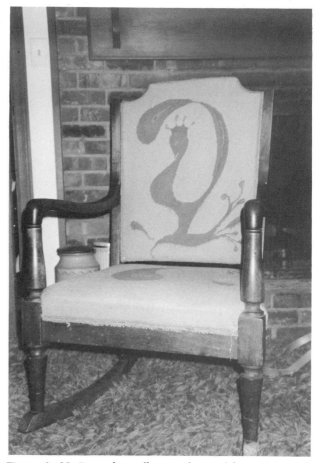

Figure 6-31. Peacock needlepoint designed for antique rocking chair, by author.

smallest and largest forms of this work (Fig. 6-31). Needlepoint can be done in continental or diagonal stitches, which appear identical on the surface, but differ in method. These are often used to produce flowers, landscapes, and other such designs. Crewel stitches also can be adapted to canvas.

Bargello is also done on canvas skrim. The yarn is laid in vertical stitches covering several horizontal threads forming colorful geometric designs (Fig. 6-32).

CASE EXAMPLES

Jane G., an 84-year-old homemaker, sustained a fracture of the trochanter of the left femur while preparing a meal at home. Since the surgical reduction of the fracture, she has exhibited signs of dementia. Her earlier interests in knitting and crocheting are too complex for her at the present time, and she has limitations in vision caused by developing cataracts.

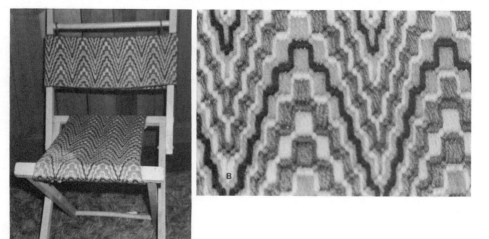

Figure 6-32. Bargello child's beach chair and detail, by author.

GOALS

1. Increase upper-extremity strength.
2. Improve self-image.
3. Improve spatial orientation.
4. Develop compensatory techniques for visual deficits.

ACTIVITIES

Yarn winding, frame weaving with fringe edges.

Mrs. G. was initially given yarn to wind into balls. She was then offered a wooden frame weaving project. The yarn was precut to length. The loom was warped with alternately contrasting yarn that was also of different textures. The loom was placed in a vertical position so she would need to elevate her arms higher as each row progressed. The therapist worked closely with her to develop the concepts of over and under, while emphasizing reliance on tactile recognition. With practice she became able to work with greater accuracy and less supervision. She continued working on these projects following her cataract surgery and began to create interesting colorful designs. Several staff members brought in yarn and Mrs. G. made the yarn into pillows for them.

Ronald F., a 22-year-old, has been mentally retarded since birth. His mother and father were 45 and 58, respectively, when Ronald was born. His father died 3 years ago, at which time his mother became very concerned about her son's future. She recognized that he would outlive her and that it was time to find a home for him. Their therapist advised them that placement in a group home would be easier if Ronald were able to care for himself and assume chores in a home environment.

GOAL

1. Improve self-care skills toward independence in group living environment.

ACTIVITY

Clothing repair.

Ronald was evaluated for self-care skills. He was found to be independent in dressing and bathing. He practiced preparing simple meals with supervision. In addition, the therapist instructed Ronald in the simple sewing techniques needed to repair seams, buttons, and hems. He practiced these skills under the supervision of his mother until he was quite proficient. He was accepted into a group home within the year.

Maryanne W., a 43-year-old married real estate agent, was 32 weeks pregnant with her first child when she developed hypertension and pre-eclampsia and was confined to bed for the duration of the pregnancy. She was extremely anxious. This child was conceived after 12 years of marriage, and she anticipated that this would be her only pregnancy. Diversional sedentary activities were prescribed to alleviate stress.

GOALS

1. Reduce anxiety.
2. Provide activities that will reduce patient's inclination to move about.

ACTIVITY

Knitting.

Consultation with the patient revealed that she was taught to knit as a child but does not remember how; she never had time to pursue knitting in her busy career, although she always intended to learn. It was suggested that this was probably a good time to take up this activity, and Maryanne agreed. She spent the next month and a half knitting the baby bunting that her son wore home from the hospital.

SUMMARY

Sometimes the tendency for beginners is to seek a "cookbook" that will tell them which activities to use to remediate specific conditions. Such demands are difficult to resist, but the choice of activity depends on issues other than diagnosis. Patients' personalities and motivation, therapists' favorite activities, families' needs, likes, and dislikes, and economic factors, all enter into the choices made in the clinic. These are all issues that should be taken into account, because they are fundamental to determining whether an activity is purposeful to the doer. Building competence and confidence in patients accounts for their willingness to engage in activity. Therefore, attention to the uniqueness of the individual is vital.

Activities can be used therapeutically by adapting and grading them to meet the needs of physically and mentally disabled patients of all kinds. Activity analysis is the key to determining if particular crafts are suitable for meeting patient needs. These activities can be adapted and graded to place demands on selected physical and mental capabilities so as to increase patients' competence in these areas. Careful assessment of the client is the key. Choices of activities must stem from analyses of the client's capacities and interests. From these analyses, the therapist develops goals consistent with the patient's own goals. Thus, the therapist serves as a catalyst so the patient can become the true doer and healer of himself or herself.

There are many more handcrafts than those described in this book. Many therapists continue to study crafts throughout their lives for their own pleasure and to expand their clinical skills. Books, courses, seminars, guilds, and so on, are devoted to sharing these skills. A lifetime can be spent learning these activities. One can never have too many skills, and one's skills should not be limited to handcrafts. Rather, therapists need skills in modern activities, too, so they can meet patients' needs in this modern world. To meet these needs, this book continues with modern activities that are used in the clinic.

7

Industry and Technology

The transition from folkcrafts to activities of the technologic era evolved over centuries as humans applied their expanding ideas to the materials they knew. These adaptive changes in the way people interact with the environment took place in a clear sequence. From the use of hands, tools emerged, as opposition, dexterity, and cognitive skills enabled their development. Simple tools generated more complex tools, and the inventiveness of people expanded. The invention of wheels, gears, and levers led to increasing degrees of mechanization, which varied in application from civilization to civilization. Learning to harness electricity marked the beginning of an era of rapidly accelerating industrialization and communication. These advances were further extended by developments within the petrochemical industry and, still more recently, by nuclear, electronic, laser, and other space-age developments.

Consequently, describing folkcrafts and technology as if they were separate and discontinuous is actually a false distinction. Likewise, the tendency to assume that electronics alone represent technology is mistaken. In fact, early cultures had their own technologies. Ceramics, for one, is certainly a complex technology requiring specific and accurate skills in its manufacture. Developments in technology show a gradual transition in degrees of automation.

In earliest times, the automatic aspects of activities were limited to those skills provided by the worker. A skilled worker does much of a task automatically. In fact, the ability to perform a large part of a task automatically is one way that skillfulness is determined. As technology advanced, mechanized methods of automation were devised to make work more efficient. As activities were automated, the more rapidly and efficiently they could be

performed. Human effort merged with the most sophisticated tools and materials of each era, enabling life's tasks to be performed with greatest efficiency. While much of folkcraft became automated, many objects developed within the technologic era retained the use of hand skills in their manufacture. Human beings tend to use all their tools to do the jobs they need to do, mixing them freely as they are needed.

Modern life is very different from the past. People use their skills for new and different purposes. Some of their skills are simple; some are complex. The terms "low tech" and "high tech" are used to describe differences between the simple and complex problem solving of modern life. Low-tech gadgets or devices are made from readily available materials. High tech usually refers to sophisticated applications such as those made possible by electronic or computer equipment.

Occupational therapy's low-tech solutions are demonstrated when therapists build up handles on tools, bend utensils, adapt clothing, and so on. High-tech adaptations are seen in the clinic in the form of augmentative communications systems, environmental control units, electric wheelchairs, and so on. Modern practice freely mixes low-tech and high-tech solutions to patient problems. For example, a high-tech computer can be operated by using the low-tech head wand.

This transition in degrees of automation, and the liberal use of a range of tools, is evident throughout practice. Adaptation, regardless of the tools or media used, remains the fundamental principle of occupational therapy. Society's newest tools are readily incorporated into the clinic. New materials, new technologies, and new solutions are used to resolve patient problems. Patients who cannot perform by using low-tech applications often

129

can be made functional by using the adaptations that modern invention has made available.

As society has automated its activities, the physical or mental effort necessary to perform tasks has been reduced. The same opportunities that brought society into the space age opened new worlds for disadvantaged individuals. Inventive adaptations permitted people, both able and disabled, to experience achievements not available to them by using their personal resources alone.

On the other hand, the new technologies have not been altogether beneficial. Modern technologic automation has taken people further from the direct use of the entire complement of their sensory and motor systems. As the effort required to perform tasks is reduced, so is the sensory motor feedback that such effort provides. The natural tendency of people to do things the easy way, the same tendency that provokes human beings to create ways to make things easier for themselves, can produce a society of "couch potatoes," this author among them. The healthy activity now sought by using stylized exercise programs and conscious effort was previously an integral part of life's tasks. The desire to seek the most convenient methods can deprive people of the satisfaction and feelings of competence that active effort can provide.

Reintroducing effort through purposeful activity requires clinical decision-making. A therapist must strike a balance between automation and activity. For example, an electric wheelchair may deprive a disabled person of the exercise that a manual chair offers and the person needs. On the other hand, using precious and limited energy resources to push a wheelchair may reduce the amount of energy available for other important efforts. Knowing when to use these modern tools is as important as knowing how. Assessing an individual's goals, needs, and energy level is essential in this decision-making process.

These decisions only can be made if one knows what the options are. Keeping pace with the tools of practice is a therapist's responsibility, as is their maintenance and repair. Learning to use the tools and materials required for these activities will round out the skills needed for clinical competence. Once these skills are acquired, they can be applied therapeutically, either by teaching them to patients, preparing adaptive aids, using them to keep equipment in good condition, or documenting clinical events.

This section focuses on activities made possible through the rapid advances of mechanization, showing their application to practice. It begins where the description of handcrafts left off, showing how the craft of sewing was mechanized. It also describes how hand skills and mechanization are used together for other modern activities, including high-tech applications common to modern society. All of these applications are currently used in one area of practice or another.

MACHINE SEWING

Times and Events

Almost anything produced by hand can be made more rapidly by machine. No longer is the simple sewing needle the primary tool of the trade. With the invention of the sewing machine, many significant changes took place in the home and in industry. As the time needed to produce clothing and furnishings was reduced, so was the need for individuals to produce their own things. As people's wardrobes and decor expanded, their means of expression expanded as well.

With the speed offered by machines, mass production and distribution became possible (Fig. 7–1). The sewing machine evolved from the treadle-operated machine to the electrically driven machine, to modern computerized machines used at home and in industry. These adaptations contributed to the establishment of a major industry marked by specialization, assembly lines, and other changes in labor practices.

The origins of the labor movement in this country are often associated with the needle industry, stemming in part from the infamous Triangle Shirtwaist Company fire in New York City, in 1911, where many factory workers were killed. Concerns for worker safety that arose from this tragedy were mirrored by the concerns for workers' health and safety expressed by several founders of the profession. The needle trade is only one industry for which these concerns are relevant.

George Barton (Fig. 7–2) and Isabel Gladwin Newton Barton, two founders of the National Society for the Promotion of Occupational Therapy in 1917, devoted themselves to the rehabilitation of disabled workers in a sheltered workshop called Consolation House at Clifton Springs, New York (Fig. 7–3). George Barton believed that industrial injuries would have a greater impact on practice than the war, which was instrumental in formulating the profession at that time. His prediction was well founded. The implications of changing technologies for the health of the individual worker were of interest at the outset of the profession and remain of interest today.

> The health and safety of the worker are significant issues for current practice. Industrial accidents and work-related health problems, such as repetitive motion injuries, are modern practice concerns. Opportunities for practice in these areas continue to expand. Becoming familiar with industrial and technologic tools prepares one to understand patients' problems and experiences.

Continued on page 132

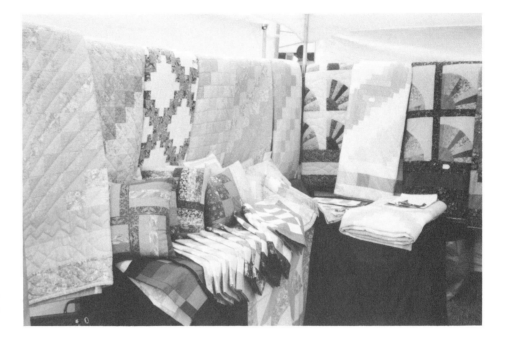

Figure 7–1. Machine-sewn needle crafts exhibited at Peters Valley, NJ, artist unknown.

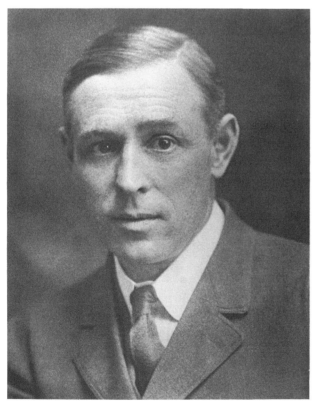

Figure 7–2. "It is improbable that more will be crippled at the front than suffer annually from accidents in industry." George Barton, 1919. (Courtesy of *OT Week*.)

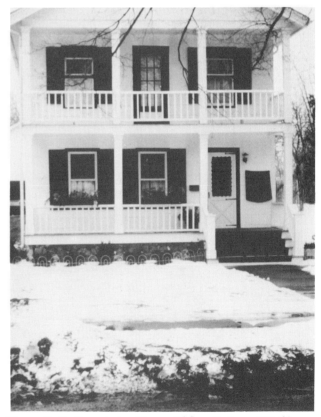

Figure 7–3. Consolation House, Clifton Springs, NY. (Courtesy of *OT Week*.)

Aside from these issues, sewing is a skill that may be used as a therapeutic activity with some patients. Furthermore, its clinical value to therapists extends beyond its use as a therapeutic activity for patients. Sometimes it is necessary to design or adapt articles of clothing and other items made of cloth or leather such as splints and walker or wheelchair bags. Competence in the use of a sewing machine is a vital skill for practice, because it enables therapists to develop and adapt such items readily.

Doll

Making a doll is a simple project of almost universal appeal from which many sewing skills can be learned.

Pattern Designing

Patterns can be traced from items from which the seams have been opened with a stitch ripper. However, most commonly, patterns are purchased at fabric stores and specialty shops where they are available in every size and description. Simple patterns also can be made from drawings or tracings, which can be enlarged by transferring the drawing or tracing to graph paper where each unit of the graph equals a larger unit.

You will need:

Newspaper or kraft paper
Graph paper (optional)
Chalk or crayon
Scissors
Straight pins

1. Design a pattern.
2. Trace the pattern onto newspaper or kraft paper.
3. Add seam allowances of ⅝ inch around the perimeter of each pattern piece.
4. Cut on the line

Cutting the Fabric

You will need:

Fabric
Pattern
Pattern marker
Tracing paper
Tracing wheel
Straight pins
Pin cushion
Scissors

1. Select a washable lightweight fabric such as cotton or polyester, or a blend of each. Solids or small prints are good for first projects. Do not choose stripes or plaids until you have some experience sewing, because these patterns must be matched, require more fabric, and are not as economical.

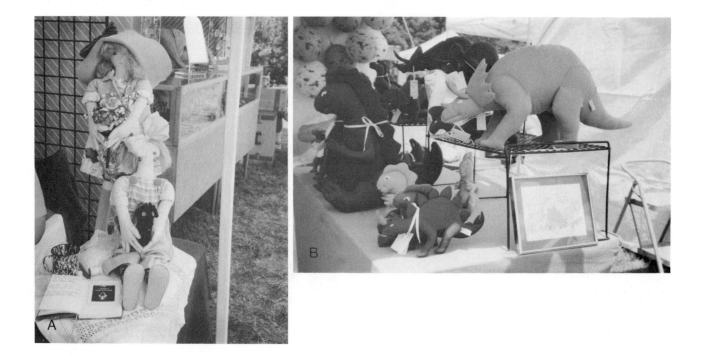

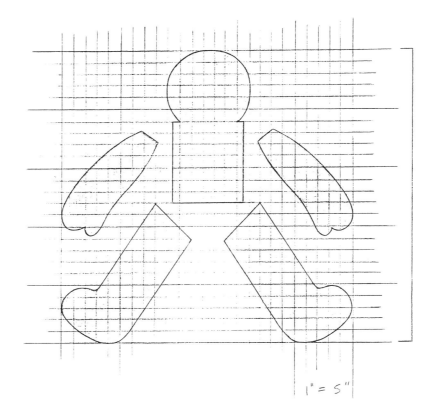

1" = 5"

2. Fold the fabric in half so the right sides of the cloth face one another.

3. Place tracing paper and pattern onto the fabric and pin in place.

4. Trace on the line with a tracing wheel. Remove tracing paper.

5. Cut on the line, yielding two identical pieces of fabric.

6. Pin the fabric pieces together so the pins lie perpendicular to the edge of the fabric with the pin heads extending off the edges of the cloth so they will not interfere with the machine needle.

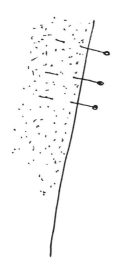

Threading the Sewing Machine

You will need:

Sewing thread
Sewing machine

A sewing machine must be threaded precisely. Many machines have a diagram imprinted on them that shows each point where the machine must be threaded. If the diagram is not on the machine, look in the manual. Follow the threading sequence exactly, because each style of sewing machine is different. Sewing machines have bobbins as well as needles. The bobbin is a small round metal or plastic unit wound with thread. It sits in a well beneath the foot plate where the sewing needle enters. The sewing machine is designed to engage the needle and bobbin threads between each stitch. Follow bobbin winding instructions from the manual precisely, because different brands of sewing machines are designed differently. Careful reading of the manual prior to use is strongly recommended to avoid unnecessary confusion.

1. Sewing machine needles are designed so the eye is at the bottom and the shaft at the top. The shaft is rounded on one side and flat on the other. Face the correct side of the shaft toward you according to the directions. Insert the needle into the fitting. Tighten the screw that holds the needle in place.

2. Follow the threading diagram on the sewing machine or in the manual. Thread the needle from front to back.

3. Wind the bobbin with thread according to the manual. Slide the footplate aside and drop the bobbin in place.

4. Hold the bobbin thread clear and slide the foot plate closed.

5. Hold the needle and bobbin threads taut.

6. Lower the needle manually by turning the wheel toward you. Continue turning the wheel toward you and the needle will raise. When the needle returns to the upright position, the bobbin and needle threads will be entwined.

7. Draw both threads toward you about 12 inches.

Sewing

You will need:

Fabric
Sewing thread
Sewing machine
Scissors

1. Place the fabric so that the seam allowance lies to the right of the needle, and the rest of the fabric is on the left. While the seam allowance for most sewing is ⅝ inch, a doll requires only ⅜ inch.

2. Lower the needle so it pierces the fabric* at the seam line.

3. Lower the foot to hold the fabric in place.

4. Stitch in reverse for 1 or 2 stitches.

5. Once the reverse stitches are made, place the machine in the forward position and press the sewing machine pedal or knee control to activate the machine.

6. Sew a seam around the perimeter, leaving a 3-inch opening. When turning a corner, stop sewing with the needle remaining in the cloth. Raise the foot to turn the fabric; lower it to resume sewing.

7. To end the seam, stitch in reverse for 1 or 2 stitches to secure the stitches. Cut the thread.

Finishing

You will need:

Sewing thread
Scissors
Straight pins
Pin cushion
Stuffing (fiberfill or cut-up nylon stockings)

1. Being careful not to cut through the seam lines, snip the fabric on the concave and convex edges of curves to keep the fabric from bunching or pulling.

*Beginners may want to practice on a piece of paper on which straight and curved lines are drawn before sewing on the fabric. When using paper, practice without threading the machine.

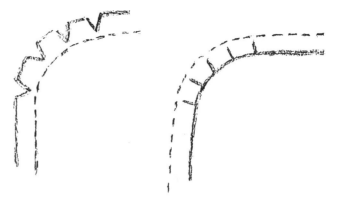

2. Snip hanging threads close to the fabric.
3. Turn inside out.
4. Stuff firmly with polyester fiberfill or with cut-up nylon stockings.
5. Turning under the rough edges, pin the opening closed and hand stitch.
6. Decorate and dress the doll as you like.

> Do not use buttons to decorate children's dolls and toys because they can come loose and children can put them in their mouths where they can be swallowed or become lodged in their windpipes. Use nontoxic paints, yarn, felt or embroidery floss for decoration.

These same techniques can be used to create pillows, clothing, and many other items. Other useful techniques are setting a zipper, doing machine-made hems, and making buttonholes. These and many other techniques can be learned as your interests in sewing and tailoring expand.

CASE EXAMPLE

Laura G. is a 32-year-old married woman with three children, 5, 6, and 8 years of age. She is an active volunteer in her children's school and is a committed homemaker.

After several months of increasing irritability, exhaustion, and lethargy, all of which she and her family attributed to her demanding schedule, Laura experienced an acute episode of illness. Following school one day, her children found her unresponsive on the kitchen floor. They called their father in his office who notified the emergency squad. Laura was taken to the hospital where she was diagnosed as a diabetic and placed on an insulin regimen. The physician referred her to a dietitian for nutritional counseling and to an occupational therapist for evaluation of her activity schedule. Consultation with Laura revealed that she was concerned about costs that would be incurred for her family as a result of her illness. She was also concerned that she might need to limit the time she would spend on school trips and other events and that this would make her children feel deserted. Laura revealed that she had always been interested in learning to sew but had never had the time because of her busy schedule.

GOALS

1. Energy conservation through alternative homemaking methods.

2. Redirect parenting activities within limits imposed by variations in energy levels.

3. Generate moderate source of income to supplement family needs.

4. Increase leisure skills.

ACTIVITY

Learn to use the sewing machine and follow patterns.

Laura learned to use the sewing machine by making simple toys and then clothes for her children. They were very pleased with their special gifts and Laura felt satisfied that she was still giving them the attention she wanted to offer. As she became adept at sewing, she found several patterns in magazines that were very appealing. She found that she could cut several patterns at one time and produce a number of projects at once. She began to use these items as gifts, and she placed some of her work in a community consignment shop. By cutting costs and generating income in this way, she applied these funds to purchase help for labor-intensive homemaking chores, thereby stabilizing her energy output and sustaining consistent and functional blood sugar levels.

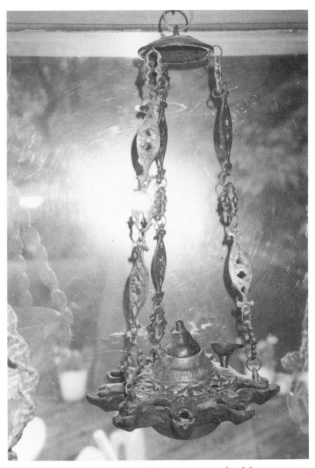

Figure 7–4. Antique brass ceremonial oil lamp.

METALWORK

Times and Events

The ability to work metal came with the ability to generate and control heat. As these skills were refined, they were adapted to the manufacturing of limitless items. The durable nature of metals and its many uses contributed to the development of civilization.

Bronze Age metals, including copper, silver, and gold, appear among ancient artifacts. These metals were worked into ornamental pieces that remain as beautiful today as when they first were made (Fig. 7–4). The choices of materials increased over time, expanding metal artistry and function. Some ancient designs are the basis for jewelry made by modern artisans.

The Iron Age ushered in a new era that changed life to an extraordinary degree. Iron was worked into tools, weapons, structures, and art forms (Figs. 7–5 and 7–6). Industrialization evolved, largely enabled by the use of metal for building machinery and the structures in which

to house them. Still later, the development of steel and other alloys brought us into the modern age, enabling advances in construction, mechanization, medicine, and many other technologies.

Aside from its potential use in therapeutic activities therapists use metal to fabricate splints and other adaptive equipment. Therefore, developing skill in the manipulation of metal expands therapists' capabilities in several directions. The dexterity needed to manipulate metal is a useful skill that can be applied to many clinical purposes. The dexterity gained in working metal may be used to adjust wheelchair parts and modify other adaptive equipment.

Copper is a practical material with which to begin to learn to work metal. It is easily malleable, and, compared with precious metals, its price is reasonable. Attractive objects can be made with some practice.

When working with copper and other metals, be careful of foil edges and metal slivers because they are very sharp and can cut one easily.

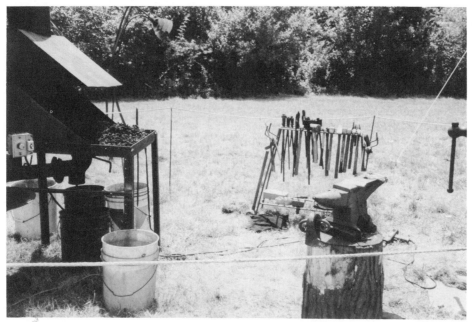

Figure 7–5. Iron worker's tools.

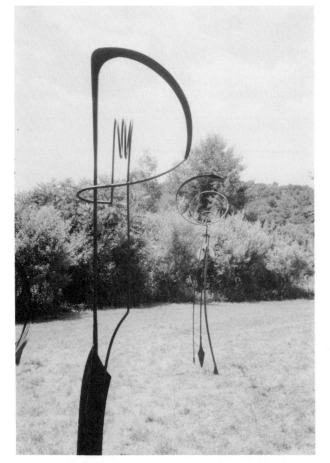

Figure 7–6. Iron sculptures, artist unknown.

Copper Tooling or Repoussé

Attractive copper foil pictures can be made by using a mold or by working free style.

Mold-Formed Copper Tooling

You will need:

Copper foil
Repoussé mold
Masking tape
Tooler or orangewood stick
Metal shears

1. Plastic molds are available in a number of designs. Select a design that you like.
2. Using metal shears, cut a piece of foil ½ inch wider and longer than the mold.
3. Place the foil on the mold, wrapping the edges of the foil around the back of the mold.
4. Turn the mold to the back and cover the edges of the foil with masking tape.
5. Press the foil with a tooler of orangewood stick until the design appears.
6. Follow directions for antiquing and mounting.

Antiquing

You will need:

Liver of sulfur
Steel wool

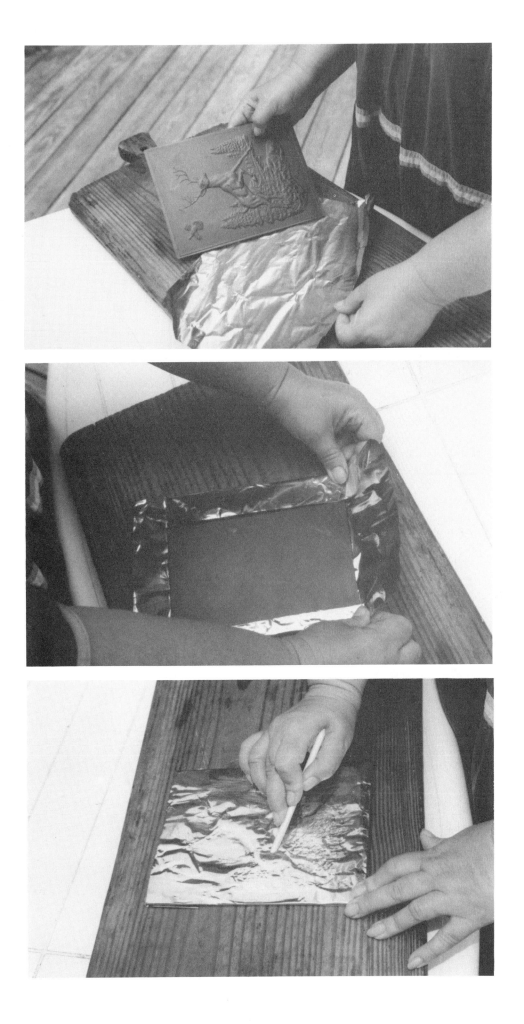

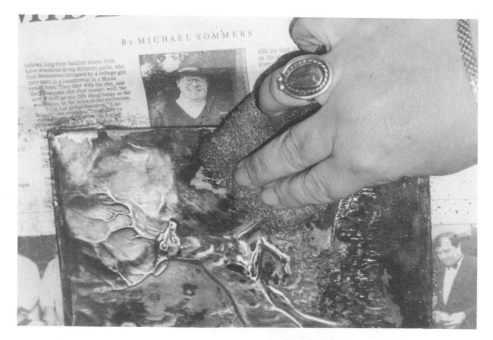

1. Turn the copper reverse side up.

2. Fill in the raised areas with plasticene modeling clay.

3. Apply liver of sulfur, a liquefied form of sulfur dioxide, to the face side. Its smell is reminiscent of rotten eggs, so be prepared for the unpleasant odor. Liver of sulfur comes in liquid or solid form. It must be used as a liquid; therefore, if it is solid, add water and mix according to manufacturer's directions. *Work in a well-ventilated area.* Moisten a cloth with liver of sulfur. Rub the cloth over the face of the picture until the copper darkens. This dark finish is called antiquing.

4. Use a fine steel wool pad to remove the antiquing selectively. Highlight the most prominent aspects of the design. The antiquing gives the design greater dimension.

Mounting on Plaques

Copper foil pictures are attractive when mounted on wooden plaques.

You will need:

Wooden plaque
Stain
Varnish
Awl
Hammer
Escutcheon pins
Acrylic spray

1. Finish the wood with stain or varnish. Allow the finish to dry before attaching the copper.

2. Place the picture on the wood.

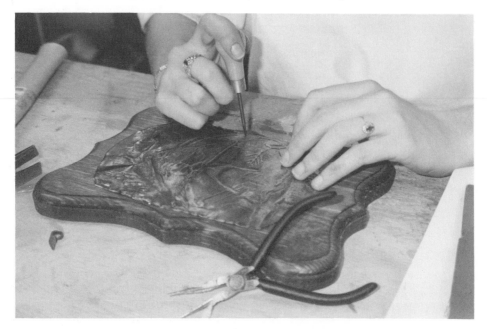

2. Using metal shears, cut a piece of foil ½ inch longer and wider than the picture you have chosen.

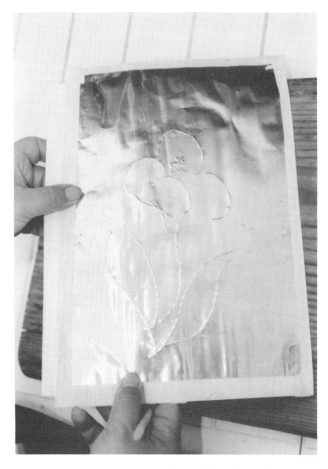

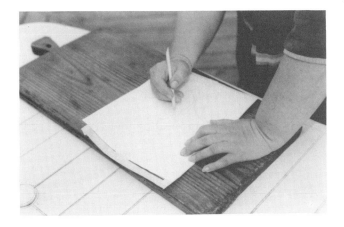

3. Use an awl to pierce the copper and wood approximately ⅜ inch in from the edges.

4. Secure the 4 corners with escutcheon pins. Continue setting the escutcheon pins evenly around the edges, approximately every ⅜ inch.

5. Spray the plaque with acrylic to keep it from tarnishing.

Free-Form Copper Tooling

You will need:

Copper foil
Masking tape
Tooler or orangewood stick
Metal shears

1. Draw or select a design that appeals to you.

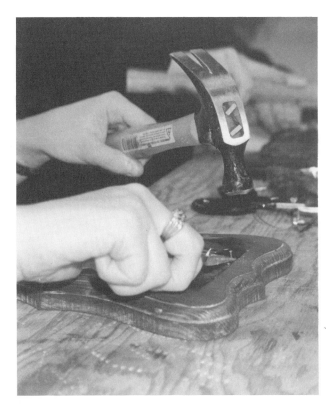

3. Bind the sharp edges of the foil with masking tape.

4. Tape the design onto the copper and scribe it into the foil with a tooler or an orangewood stick, working on a firm surface such as a table top.

5. Remove the pattern.

6. Turn the copper onto the reverse side. Place it on a thick stack of newspapers or felt pad.

7. With the flattened end of the tooler, press down into selected areas to raise the design.

8. Place the copper face up on a firm surface. You will see that a bas-relief design has emerged. Press the background flat to make the design appear in greater relief.

9. Continue reversing from front to back until you are satisfied with the appearance of your work. Fill the back with plasticene.

10. Finish with liver of sulfur and mount or frame.

> The grasp used to hold the tooler is identical to that used in writing, so copper tooling is a good prewriting task and can be used to transfer hand dominance. Working copper free-form requires more skill and creativity than using a mold and takes more time to complete.

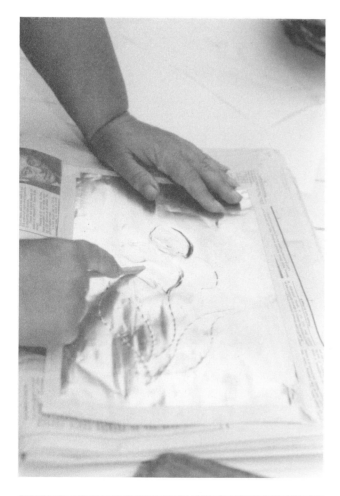

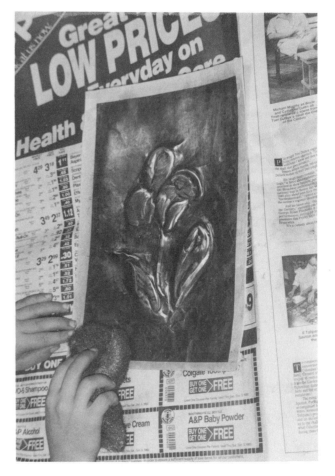

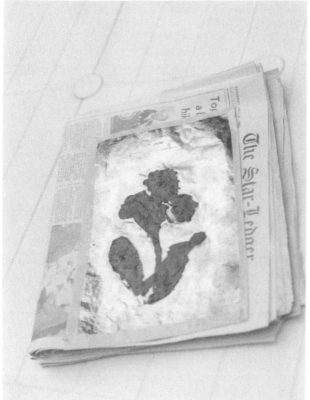

Enameling

Enameling on copper is used to produce earrings, pins, paintings, and other beautiful objects (Fig. 7–7). Blanks of copper are commercially available, although any shape can be cut from copper sheeting with a jeweler's saw and filed smooth with a jeweler's file.

You will need:

Copper blanks
Steel wool
Enamel
Enameling kiln (Fig. 7–8)
Gum of tragacanth
Earring and pin backs
Glue

1. Lightly rub the copper with fine steel wool.
2. Spread a thin coating of gum of tragacanth onto the copper.
3. Sprinkle colored enamel onto the copper, creating a design of your liking.
4. Fire in an enameling kiln, following the manufacturer's instructions.
5. Glue on pin or earring backs, or frame.

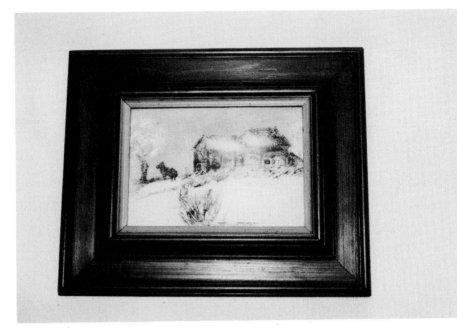

Figure 7–7. Enamel on copper, by Lenore Breslaw.

This task requires precision in fine motor skills. The temperature of the kiln and objects heated can cause burns, so precautions must be taken. Place objects to cool on a heat-resistant surface back from the work area.

Wire Jewelry

Wire can be bent into interesting shapes to make necklaces, bracelets, and earrings. The pattern shown is similar to one by ancient South American artisans on exhibit at the American Museum of Natural History in New York City.

You will need:

Copper wire, 16 or 18 gauge
Needle-nose half-round pliers
Wire cutter
Liver of sulfur
Steel wool

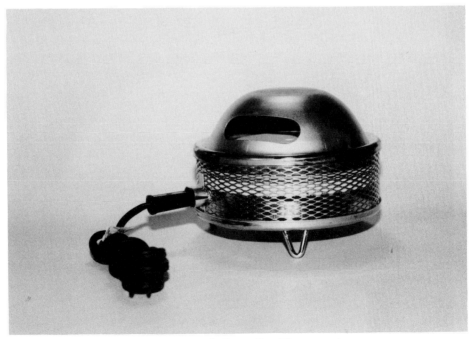

Figure 7–8. Enameling kiln.

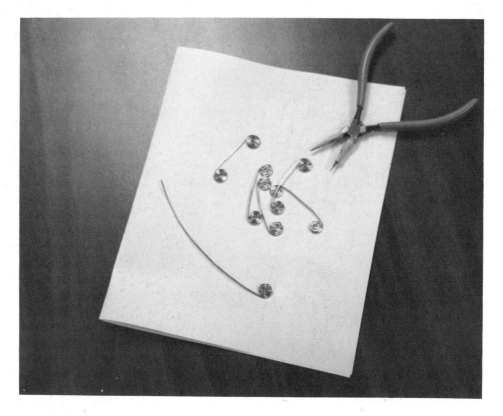

1. For the bracelet, cut 18 pieces of wire, 6½ inches in length. Cut one piece of wire 7½ inches long, to be used as the hook for fastening. The necklace requires 32 pieces of wire.

2. Using needle-nose pliers, grasp the end of one piece of wire with the tip of the pliers, bending it so as small a loop as possible is created. Hold the loop with the pliers and wrap the rest of the wire tightly around the loop into a coil. Repeat on the opposite end of the wire, creating a link with coils on each end. You may wish to wrap the pliers with masking tape to prevent marking the wire.

3. Repeat with each piece of wire.

4. Bend each link precisely in the center, forming a loop.

5. Fold the loop over, completing a link.

6. Interlock the links.

7. Wrap a short length of wire around a round pencil or dowel rod. Slip the wire off the pencil. Clip with wire cutters to form links. Add to the first link of the bracelet.

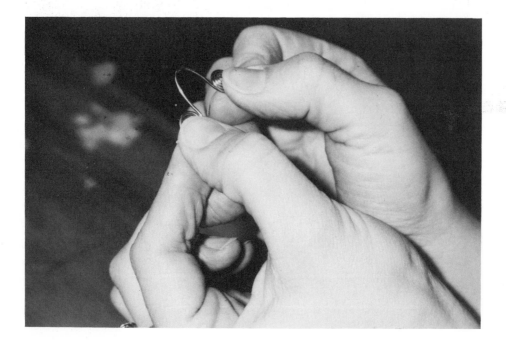

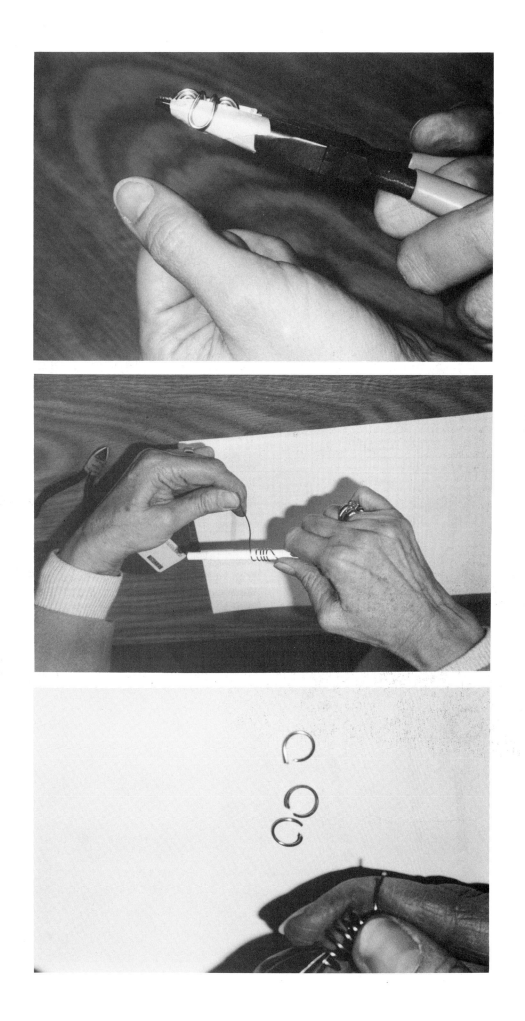

8. Close the link by pressing the ends sideways toward each other.

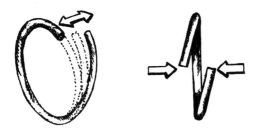

9. Add the 7½-inch link to the last link, finishing the bracelet.

10. You may antique the bracelet by applying liver of sulfur, or you may apply colorless nail polish to retain the shiny finish of the copper wire.

This same design also can be made into earrings. With some experimentation, other designs and objects can be made.

> This task is bilateral, repetitive, and time-consuming. Completing it requires hand strength and precision.

CASE EXAMPLE

F.J., a 42-year-old machinist, developed a sarcoma of the distal end of the left humerus, necessitating an above-the-elbow amputation. F.J. was married with two teenage sons. He was depressed about his appearance and his potential to resume his occupation but was motivated to return to work.

GOALS

1. Prevocational training.
2. Increase bilateral upper-extremity skills using an above-elbow hook prosthesis.
3. Improve feelings of self-efficacy and self-image.

ACTIVITY

Wire jewelry.

F.J. was introduced to wire jewelry as a task that would require precise use of his prosthesis. The use of the steel hook could substitute for pliers, and the skills he learned would compare to those he used on the job. F.J. completed a necklace, bracelet, and earrings, which he gave to his wife. Having successfully completed this activity, his feelings about his competence improved and he was encouraged to accept job retraining that enabled him to return to work. He was provided with a cosmetic hand, which he used when he was not at work.

WOODWORKING

Times and Events

Wood is a readily available natural material obtained from trees. Depending on its source, it is light or heavy, hard or soft, durable or fragile (Table 7–1). Wood has been transformed into a multitude of items of great usefulness and beauty in every era since ancient times. (Figs. 7–9 through 7–13). Selecting the correct material is determined by the use to which the item is to be put.

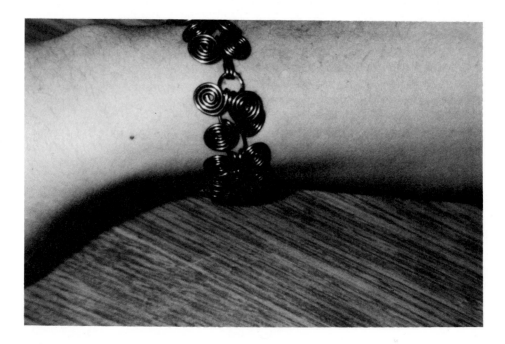

Table 7–1. SOME COMMONLY USED WOODS
AND THEIR CHARACTERISTICS

Cherry—light brown or red. Medium hardness and
    strength. Use for furniture. Usually rubbed and
    polished.
Mahogany—red or brown. Medium hardness and
    strength. One of the best furniture woods. Finish
    without stain.
Maple—red. Hardwood, strong. One of the best
    hardwoods.
Oak—red or white. Hardwood. Pores are very open.
    Stains well, shows grain.
Pine—white. Softwood. Stains well in browns. Good
    all-purpose material. Excellent for paint.
Walnut—brown. Medium hardness. Strong. Good for
    furniture and cabinets.

Kitchen implements, houses, furniture, and model airplanes all are made from various sorts of woods.

Wood is worked with hand tools and mechanical tools. Most woodworkers use a combination of both. As modern technologies such as lasers and computers were developed, they were adapted to woodworking, but tools and techniques developed in ancient times remain as relevant to modern woodcrafters as ever. Hammers and chisels are as important to the modern woodworker as are electric drills and saws.

Woodworking has been identified traditionally as a masculine activity. Because our society still tends to differentiate some tasks of women from those of men, woodworking is largely unfamiliar to many occupational therapy students before entering school, because the majority of the students are women. Therefore, gaining competence in woodworking is a milestone for many of them. Achieving these skills enables the students to recognize similarities among many different media and tools, despite gender issues. For example, the sewing machine and jigsaw are remarkably similar tools. By divesting themselves of bias as well as the fear of saws, drills, and other mechanical and electric tools, the students take a step toward the confidence needed for practice, not to mention other life pursuits.

Whether directed toward vocational or leisure pursuits, learning to work in wood requires precision and adeptness. The number of items that can be made of wood is limitless and can meet many clinical needs. Developing skill in woodworking not only enables therapists to instruct patients in this craft, but also prepares the therapists to create adaptive equipment.

Many of the tools and skills used to work wood also can be applied to working plastics, another medium used for making adaptive equipment.

Because of the nature of modern clinics, offices, and itinerant practices, this section has been restricted to the use of portable electric and hand tools. See Table 7–2 for safety instructions for power tools.

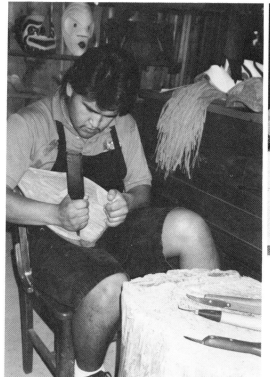

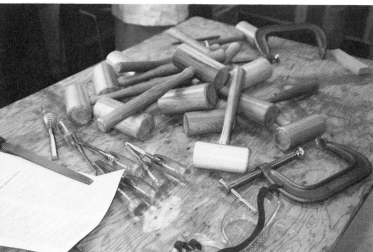

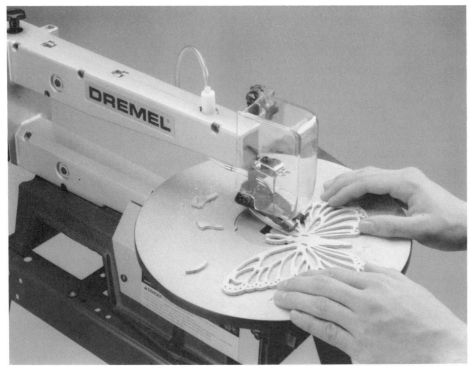

Courtesy of Dremel, Inc., Racine, WI.

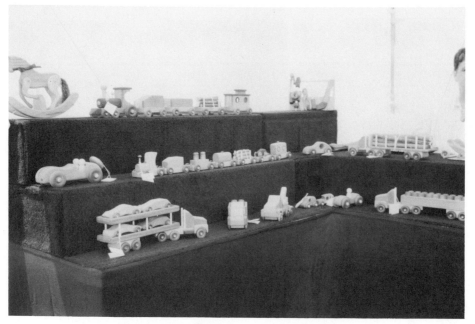

Figure 7–9. Whittled cars, artist unknown.

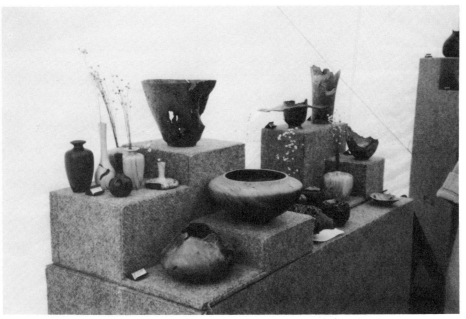

Figure 7 – 10. Wood lathed bowls, artist unknown.

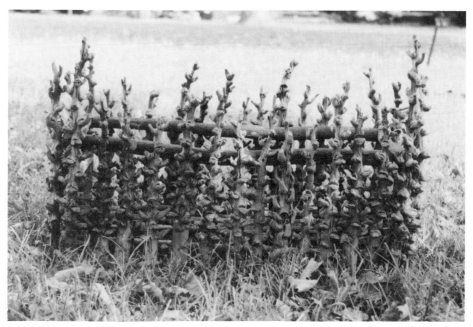

Figure 7 – 11. Olivewood twig basket from Maryland, artist unknown.

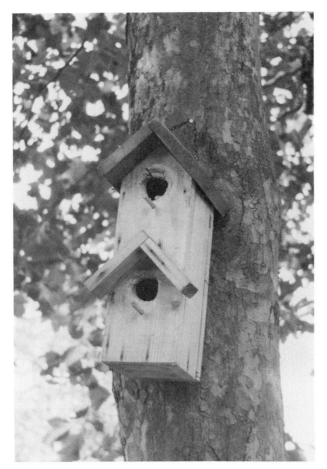

Figure 7–12. Birdhouse, artist unknown.

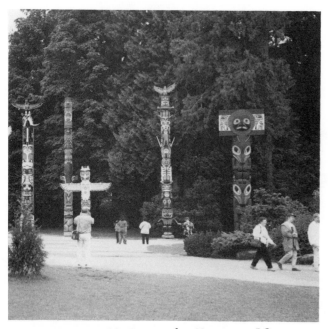

Figure 7–13. Totem poles, Vancouver, BC.

Table 7–2. SAFETY INSTRUCTIONS FOR POWER TOOLS

1. Ground all tools.

2. Keep guards in place.

3. Create a safe environment.
   Keep work area clean.
   Floor must not be slippery.
   Do not use power tools in damp or wet locations.
   Keep work area well lit.
   Provide adequate surrounding work space.

4. Keep visitors a safe distance from work area.

5. Do not force the tool.

6. Use the right tool for the job.

7. Wear the proper attire.
   Do not wear loose clothing, gloves, neckties, or
      jewelry (rings, wristwatches).
   Tie back long hair.
   Roll long sleeves above the elbow.

8. Use safety goggles

9. Use dust masks.

10. Secure work with clamps or vise.

11. Do not overreach; keep proper footing and balance.

12. Maintain tools with care.
    Sharp tools are safe tools.

13. Disconnect tools before servicing and when
    changing blades and so on.

14. Make sure switch is "off" before plugging in cord.

15. Never leave tool running unattended.
    Turn power off.
    Do not leave tool until it comes to a complete stop.

Nails and Screws

Nails and screws are manufactured for many uses. They come in graduated lengths and widths, and should be appropriate for the uses to which they are put. Each is manufactured in different styles.

Nails

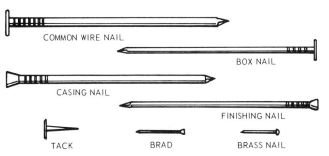

COMMON WIRE NAIL

BOX NAIL

CASING NAIL

FINISHING NAIL

TACK   BRAD   BRASS NAIL

Adapted from Craft Techniques in Occupational Therapy. Department of the Army, Washington, DC, 1980, p 12-80.

Screws

Measure the width of the boards being joined. For most uses, select a screw 1½ times as long as the depth of one board. Measure the width of the screw shaft to select the correct size drill bit.

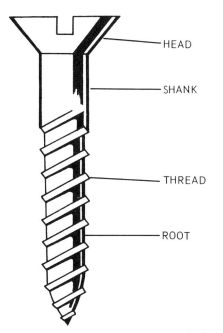

HEAD

SHANK

THREAD

ROOT

Adapted from Craft Techniques in Occupational Therapy. Department of the Army, Washington, DC, 1980, p 12-89.

Table Lamp

One project that uses a number of hand and mechanical skills is a table lamp. The same skills learned in making this lamp can be applied to making many other items useful in the clinic. This lamp was designed by Eva Siegel, OTR, especially to teach occupational therapy students these varied skills.

You will need:

Wood
Crosscut saw
Motorized table jigsaw
Electric drill
Drill bits, assorted sizes
Phillips head screwdriver
Slit head screwdriver
Clamps
Vise
Rasp
Half-round file
Sandpaper—coarse and fine
Level
Carpenter's square
Chisel
Tung oil or stain
Rags
¼-round, ¼-inch dowel (optional)
Wood glue (optional)
Brass escutcheon pins (optional)
Hammer

Sawing

1. Measure a 12 × 24 inch piece of Phillipine mahogany or other suitable lumber from a length of board. Mark across its width with a pencil and a square.
2. Place the board across two sawhorses or chairs. Cut on the line with a crosscut saw.
3. Trace the four pattern pieces onto the wood.
4. Cut out the pieces using a table jigsaw. *Wear safety goggles to protect your eyes.* Press the wood flat against the saw table. Turn on the saw. Push the wood lightly against the blade; do not push hard or twist the blade, or it may snap. Cut to the outside of the lines.

Many simple craft projects can be made by using a jigsaw (Fig. 7–14).

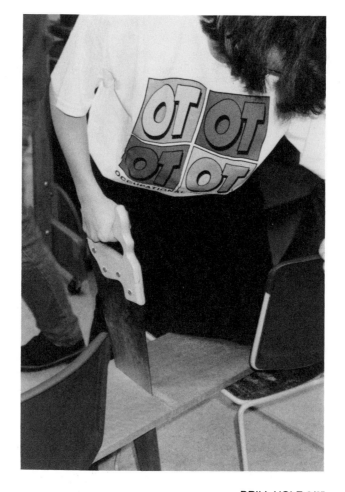

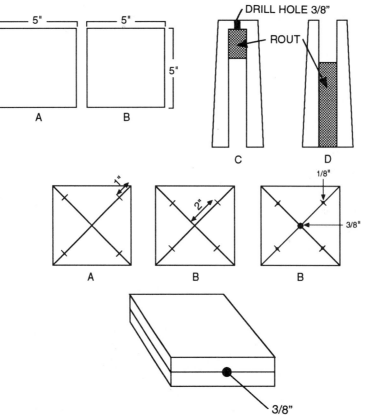

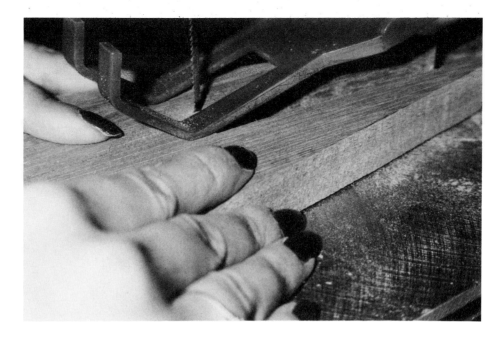

Replacing Jigsaw Blades

Breaking the blade while sawing is noisy and frightening. However, there is no cause for alarm. Learning how to replace a blade is part of becoming familiar with the saw.

1. Turn off the saw and remove the plug from the electric socket.
2. Unsnap the blade locking mechanism. Remove the broken blade.
3. Insert a new blade with the teeth facing downward and toward you. Be certain it is securely attached to the sprockets that hold it in place. Snap the locking mechanism shut.

4. Reinsert the plug into the wall.
5. Turn on the machine and continue to saw.

Filing and Sanding

1. When all the pieces are cut out, place each one in turn in a vise.
2. File the edges level and smooth, using a rasp and then a file.
3. Check the squareness of the edges with a level.
4. Sand with the grain using a sanding block, using coarse and then fine sandpaper.*

---

*When selecting sandpaper, fine sandpaper generally has a higher number than coarse, but the numbers vary among manufacturers.

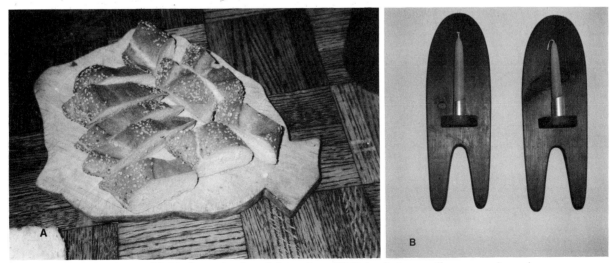

Figure 7-14. (A) Maple cutting board, by author. (B) Stained pine candle sconces, by author.

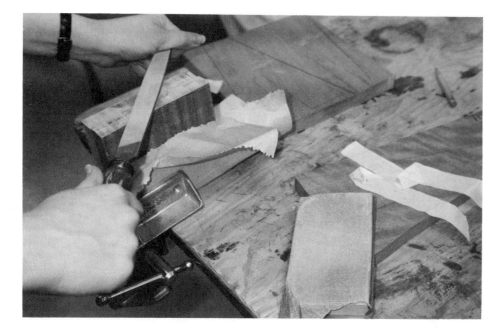

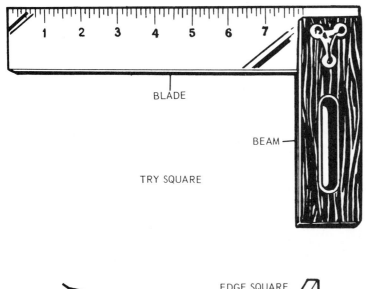

BLADE

BEAM

TRY SQUARE

From Craft Techniques in Occupational Therapy. Department of the Army, Washington, DC, 1980, p 12-45.

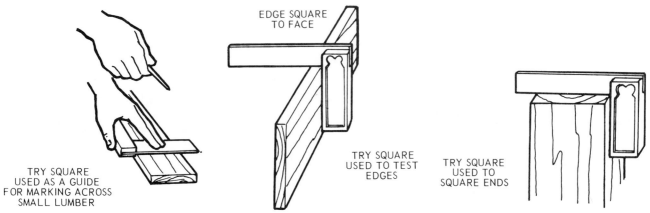

TRY SQUARE
USED AS A GUIDE
FOR MARKING ACROSS
SMALL LUMBER

EDGE SQUARE
TO FACE

TRY SQUARE
USED TO TEST
EDGES

TRY SQUARE
USED TO
SQUARE ENDS

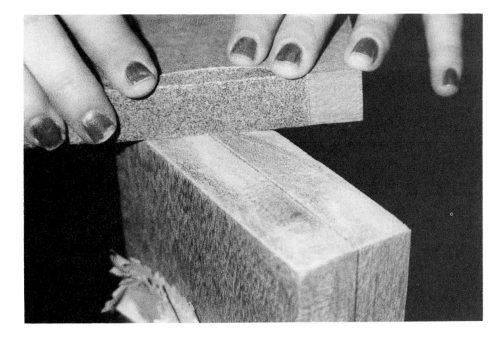

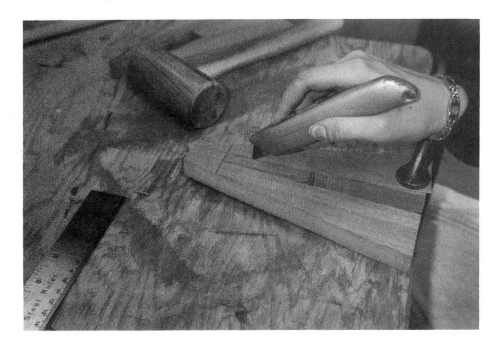

Routing

1. Draw 2 parallel lines ⅜ inch apart. Score along the lines with a knife.

2. Use a chisel and mallet to cut a channel, routing between the lines to a depth of ¼ inch.

Drilling and Assembling

1. Fit the 2 cross pieces of the lamp together.

2. Unplug the drill. Open the chuck with the key.

3. Insert the drill bit deep into the chuck and tighten it securely with the key. Insert the plug into the electric socket.

4. For the base, draw 2 diagonal lines from corner to corner on pieces A and B.

5. On piece A, mark 1 inch in from each corner.

6. Drill four ⅛-inch holes, 1 inch in from the corners.

7. On piece B, mark 2 inches in from each corner.

8. Drill four ⅛-inch holes 2 inches in from the center.

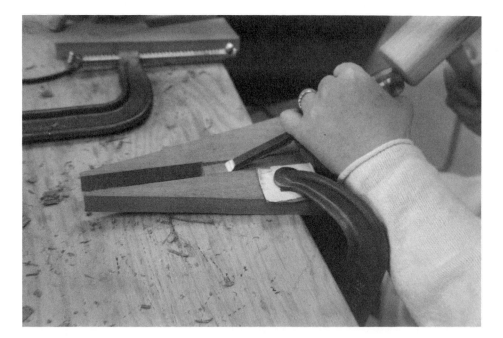

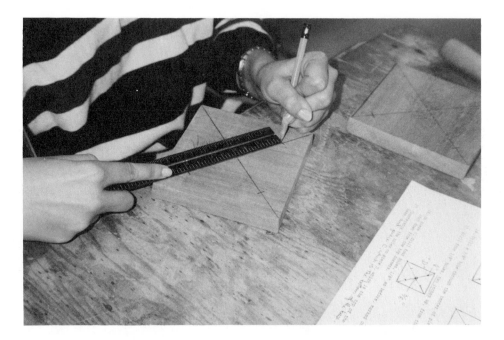

9. On piece B, drill a ⅜-inch hole through the center.

10. Countersink the holes on piece B.

11. Secure base pieces A and B together and drill a ⅜-inch hole through one end.

12. Drill a ¼-inch hole down through the top of piece C. Gouge out a small area near the top of the routed area on piece C for the lamp pipe and nut leading to the drill hole. Bevel the opening slightly to facilitate the feeding of the wire. Fit C and D together. Wire according to the directions in the section on electric wiring (see page 178).

13. Attach base B to the lamp with screws with the routed area facing toward you. Countersink the screws.

14. Clamp on base A so the sides that form the ⅜-inch hole are together; then screw pieces A and B to-

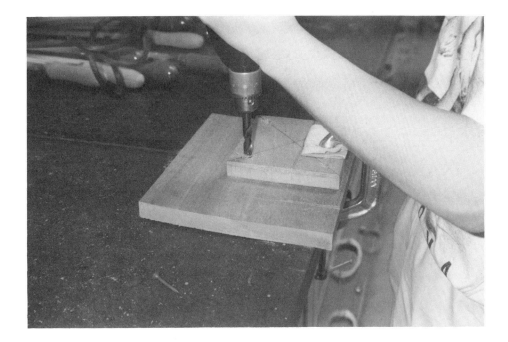

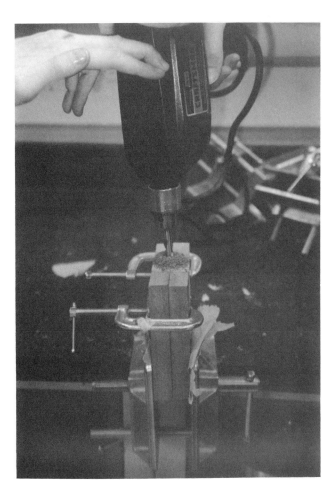

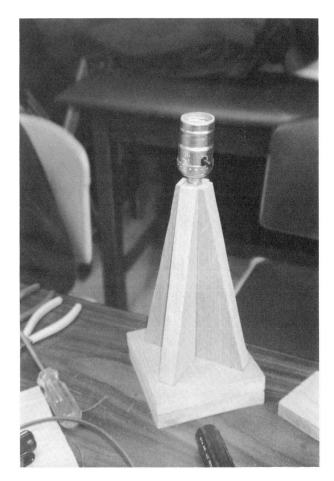

gether. Countersink the screws. The assembled lamp is shown below.

Finishing

1. Finish the wood with tung oil. Apply the oil with a rag, wait a few minutes for the oil to be absorbed, then rub off the excess. You can also stain the lamp with wood stain.

Trim (Optional)

1. Cut 4 pieces of ¼-round, ¼-inch dowel to a length of 8 inches.
2. Sand one end of each dowel until it is rounded.
3. Stain the dowels to match the lamp, or leave them natural for a contrasting look.
4. Glue in place with the flat end of the dowel at the base and the rounded end up.
5. Secure the dowels with brass escutcheon pins (optional).

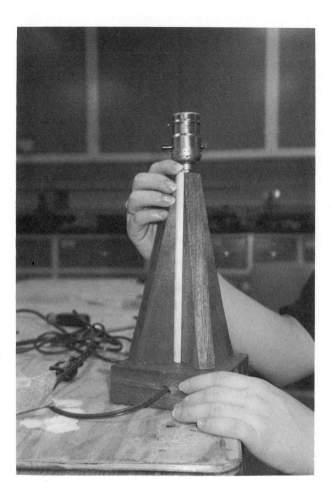

The many techniques used in completing the lamp give you the skills necessary to create most clinical adaptations such as armboards or wheelchair tray tables. These same skills can be used to make small furniture items such as book racks, shelves, birdhouses, and so on.

Kits are widely available from commercial sources and are very popular items for the clinic. The use of kits relieves therapists' time in preparation. However, be sure to use good-quality kits, or the projects will not offer the necessary positive feedback to contribute to patients' feelings of self-worth.

CASE EXAMPLE

John J., a 37-year-old divorced truck driver with a 4-year-old son, sustained multiple fractures of both femurs and right tibia in a driving accident. He was found to have been driving while intoxicated. Surgical reductions of fractures of the right lower extremity were performed, and both lower extremities were casted. A graded standing program was prescribed.

GOALS

1. Increase upper-body strength.
2. Increase standing tolerance.
3. Provide activities with strong masculine identity to reinforce feelings of competence.

ACTIVITY

Woodworking.

Woodworking was selected to meet the above stated goals and was readily accepted by the client because of his familiarity with this activity. The therapist worked with John on discharge plans. He determined that John lived alone in a sparsely furnished apartment. While John had visitation rights, he often was not sure how to relate to his young child. The therapist suggested that John might use his rehabilitation time to make something for his son such as a lamp, shelves, or a toy. He chose to make items the child could play with when he visited his father's apartment. The patient worked either at a standing table or seated in a wheelchair, increasing the standing time as his tolerance increased. The toy car and bench he made for his son were a big hit!

PAPER, PRINTING, AND PHOTOGRAPHY
Times and Events

The development of paper marked the beginning of the communications era. This durable, yet lightweight two-dimensional medium is excellent for representing, transmitting, and transporting ideas.

Paper evolved from the parchment and papyrus known in biblical times. The first paper was made from pulp materials derived from mulberry leaves and bark. This technology was developed in China and Japan and dates back to 250 BCE. Its use expanded from the Orient to the rest of the world where other materials such as linen and cotton rags were used. Modern artisans still produce handcrafted paper using rags made of natural vegetal fibers (Fig. 7–15). Commercially manufactured paper is composed primarily of wood pulp that has been processed chemically.

Developments in paper production eventually made this material readily available to the public. Its use for myriad mundane and sophisticated purposes changed people's lives in many ways. The mass production of paper led to an era of ever-increasing communication, further enabled by the automation of printing equipment, with its eventual computerization. From the biblical scribes to the production of the daily newspaper, this transition through the history of a communication me-

dium serves as a window to the development of modern civilization.

The variety of activities using paper is so broad that they are virtually unlimited. Paper can be ornamented in many ways, some simple, some complex. Here are a selection of activities that are fun to do and are useful tools for the clinic. No activities described here involve the use of a printing press, because these are not ordinarily available to modern clinicians as they once were in the past.

Paper Making

You will need:

Cotton or linen rags or newspaper
Screened frame
Wooden board
Weight (iron)
Food processor
Rectangular pan
Fabric or vegetable dye (optional)

1. Staple fine wire or nylon screening to a frame, sized so it fits into a vat or pan with room enough to shift the frame around. Standard sizes for paper are 5 × 7 inches, 8½ × 11 inches, and 11 × 14 inches. The beginner should start small. Kits are available that include screened frames.

2. Tear or cut cotton or linen rags into small pieces and soak for several hours. Or, use newspaper. Newspaper will produce darker paper.

3. Grind the rags or paper into pulp using a blender or food processor until the mix is the consistency of lumpy oatmeal.

4. Add dye or ornamental objects such as flowers, leaves, or feathers if you like.

5. Pour the pulp into the pan.

6. Submerge the frame into the pulp, covering the screen entirely.

7 As you lift the frame from the water, slosh it back and forth to spread the pulp evenly across the screen. The liquid will pass through the screen, leaving the pulp to form the paper.

8. Allow to drain or place in oven to dry at low heat.

9. Turn the paper out onto a smooth and absorbent surface such as felt, blotting paper, or newspaper covered with a clean cloth.

10. Repeat the process, layering the paper.

11. Cover the layers of paper completely with a flat board, and weight evenly until the paper has completely dried. (This may take up to 3 days.) Individual sheets may be smoothed and dried with an iron.

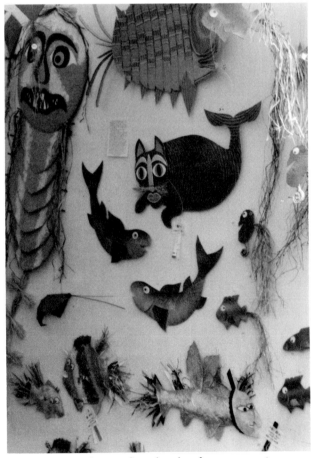

Figure 7–15. Sculptures from handmade papers, artist unknown.

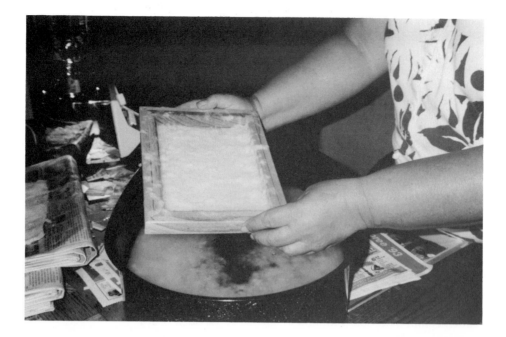

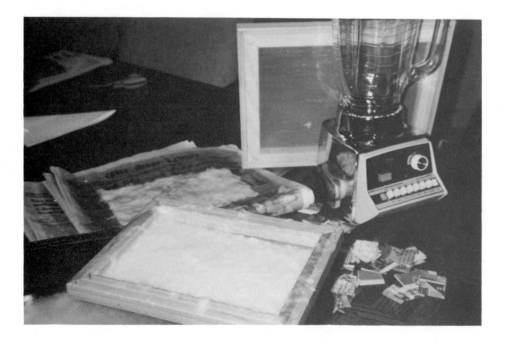

12. Clean up. Drain pulp through a mesh colander. Do not pour pulp down the drain. Squeeze out excess water. Discard, or place in plastic bags and refrigerate for up to several weeks. Add water to reconstitute.

13. The rough edges of the sheets of paper formed by this process are called a deckel edge, and they contribute to the attractiveness of handmade paper. If you prefer, the edges can be trimmed evenly by using a guillotine paper cutter.

Papier Mâché

Papier mâché is used as a sculpture medium. It is made of scraps of paper applied over a form, creating a very lightweight object that can be ornamented in many ways. It can be used to make artificial fruit, a puppet head, a sculpture, and many other objects (Fig. 7–16). Papier mâché pulp can be purchased in a powder form to which water is added, or it can be made very inexpensively of recycled newspaper.

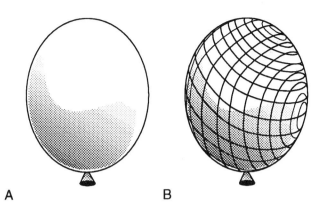

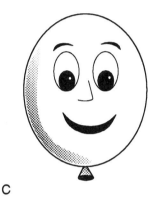

Figure 7–16. Papier mâché puppet head. (*A*) Balloon. (*B*) Balloon covered with papier mâché strips. (*C*) Balloon deflated and papier mâché painted.

You will need:

Newspaper
Flour
Oil of wintergreen
Water
Plasticene, balloon, or other form

1. Tear newspaper into 1-inch strips.
2. Prepare a solution of flour, water, and oil of wintergreen.
3. Blow up a balloon or use another shape as a base to form the object. Or plasticene can be sculpted and used as a base.
4. Dip strips of paper into the solution and apply to the form. Cover the form entirely with 3 or 4 layers.
5. Set to dry.
6. Slice in half with a sharp knife. Remove the form. Replace the halves together. Use papier mâché strips to paste the halves together.
7. Decorate with tempera paint when dry.

Greeting Cards

One simple and attractive project can be done by folding paper and dipping it into vegetable dyes of various colors. This ornamented paper can be used for notepaper, gift, wrap, greeting cards, and other such items.

You will need:

Tissue paper
Scissors
Food coloring
Freezer wrap
Electric iron
Plastic containers
Roasting pan
Guillotine paper cutter

1. Place water in several plastic containers.
2. Drop different colors of vegetable dye into each container.

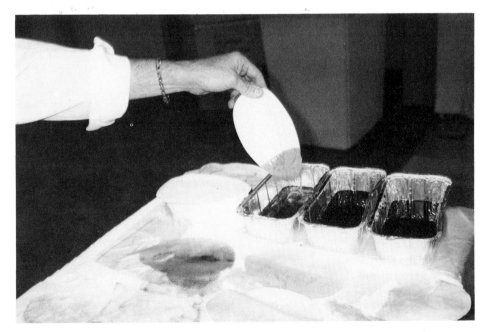

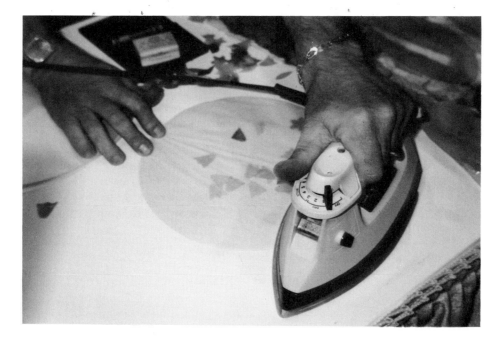

3. Fold the tissue paper several times.

4. Dip the folded tissue paper into one or more colors of your choice. The colors will bleed into the paper in interesting patterns.

5. Unfold the paper carefully, because it tends to tear when wet. Set aside to dry.

6. Place the paper on a piece of freezer wrap, shiny side up, and press with a warm iron.

7. Fold in half.

8. Trim to size with a paper cutter.

> Though this activity is very simple, some people find unfolding the tissue paper very frustrating because it tends to tear. Some patients may need help with this part of the project if they are limited in dexterity or in patience. The heat and weight of the iron may also present a problem for those with limited strength, judgment, or tactile sensitivity.
>
> Some papers have finishes that are incompatible and can interfere with one or more of the processes. Test your paper before using it in a project with patients.

Marbled Paper

Interesting and unique designs can be made by mixing paint, vegetable oil, and water together in a shallow pan and applying the mixture to paper. This technique can be used for bookbinding, gift paper, and stationery.

You will need:

Paper
Tempera paints
Vegetable oil
Aluminum pan

1. Fill aluminum pan with water to 1 inch from the top of the pan.

2. Drop 1 Tbs. of oil onto surface of colored water.

3. Stir the liquid to create swirls.

4. Touch the underside of the paper onto the surface of the water and lift off.

5. Set the paper to dry.

Matching envelopes can be made by folding a sheet of paper as shown in the accompanying figure and glueing the edges.

> This simple activity requires brief attention and results in an attractive product that is appealing to both adults and children.

Paper Folding

The art of paper folding was brought to remarkable heights by the Japanese in their art form, origami. Traditional origami does not use scissors or tape. The artistry comes from the intricate folding of paper alone. However, some attractive designs are made by cutting in addition to folding. Paper folding appeals to children and adults alike.

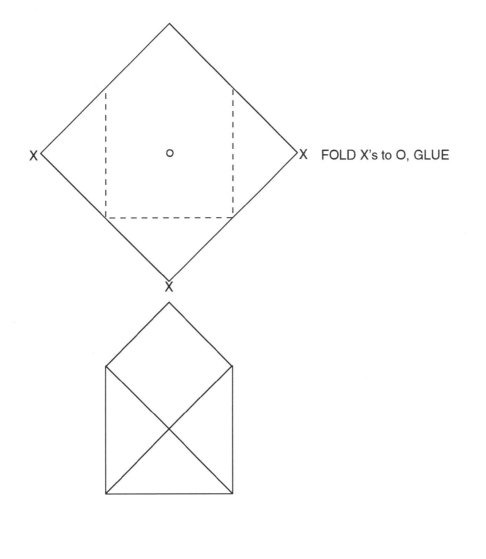

X   o   X   FOLD X's to O, GLUE

X

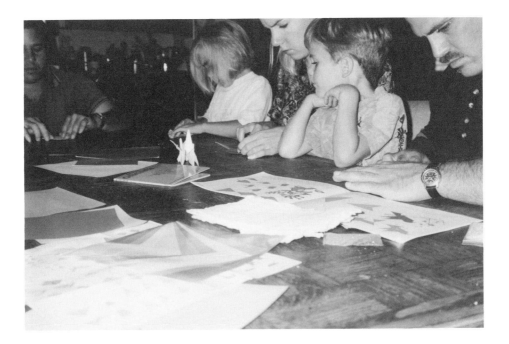

All origami projects begin with a sheet of square paper. Commercial origami paper comes already squared in various sized sheets; it usually comes with directions for a number of projects. This paper is ideal for folding because it creases cleanly and does not tear easily. When using other paper, square it by folding it on the diagonal. Cut the excess away.

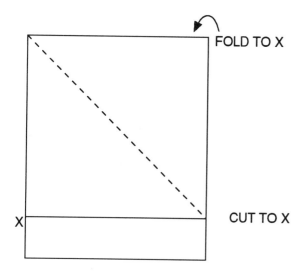

FOLD TO X

CUT TO X

X

Making party hats and paper boats is a great favorite of children and a fun activity for parties. Party hats and paper boats can be made of newspaper or newsprint, which can also be colored with crayons or tempera paints.

Party Hat

You will need:

Newspaper
Scissors
Cellophane tape

1. Fold a full sheet of paper in half at the crease. (For hat, use tabloid-sized newspaper.)
2. At the center, fold the paper on a diagonal on each side.
3. Fold 1 sheet 1½ inches up from the bottom.
4. Turn the project over to the reverse side and fold to match the first side.
5. Fold in the corners and crease sharply.

Paper Boat

1. Make the party hat described above, using 8½ × 11 inch paper.
2. Open it wide and fold along the alternate dimension.
3. Fold each side in half, bringing the bottom point up to the top point on each side.
4. Spread the outer points apart, pulling the edges into a straight line.
5. This can be decorated with watercolor paints. This boat will actually float in water!

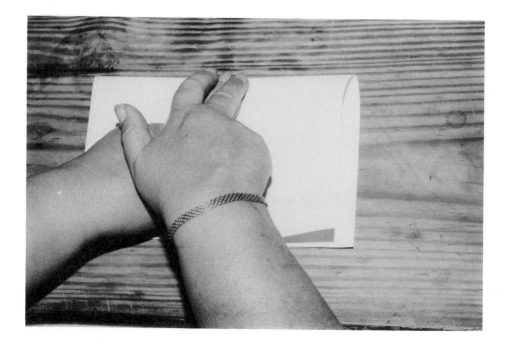

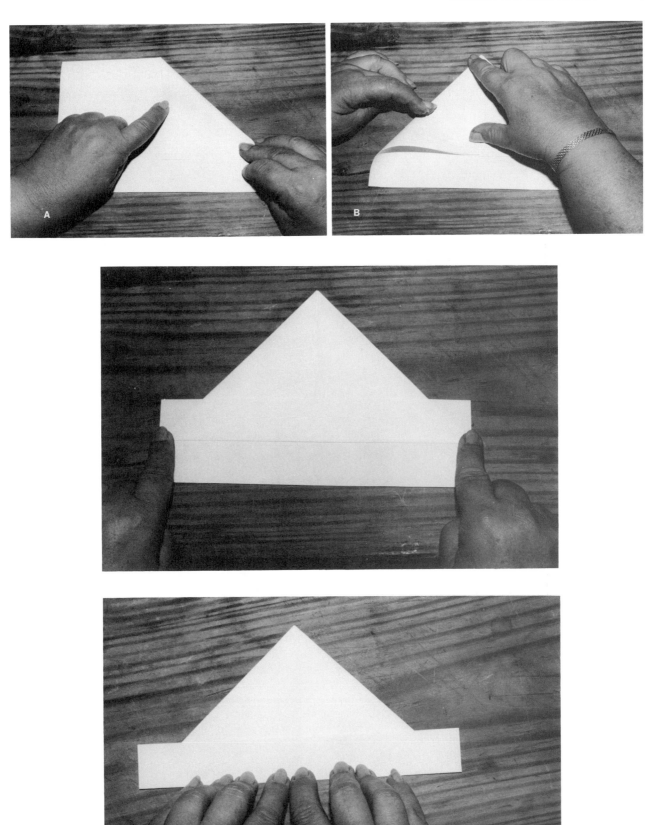

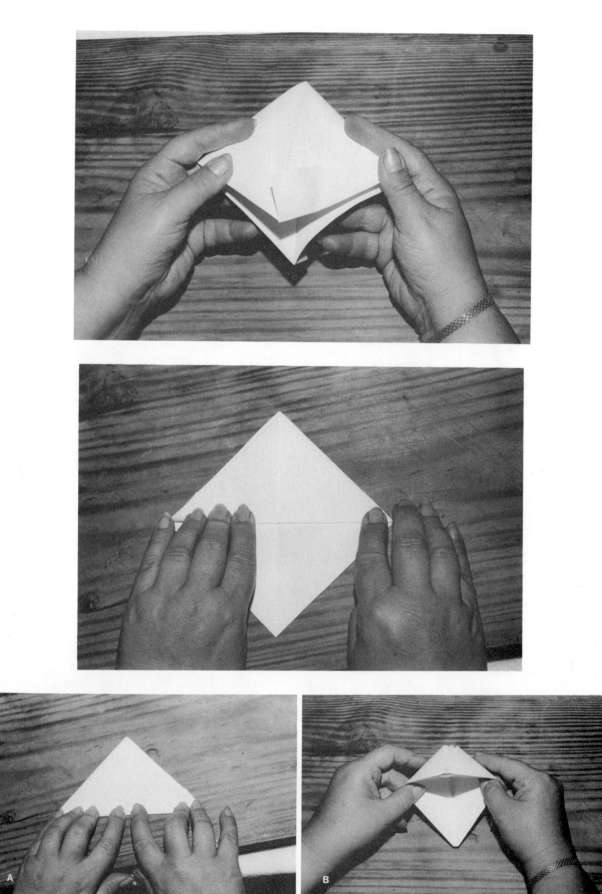

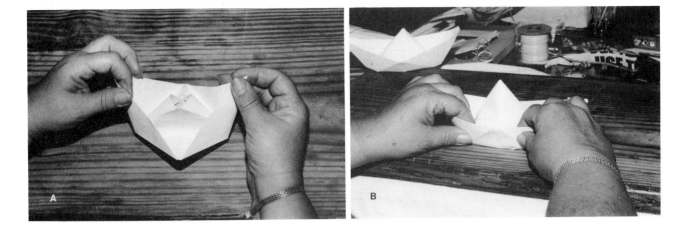

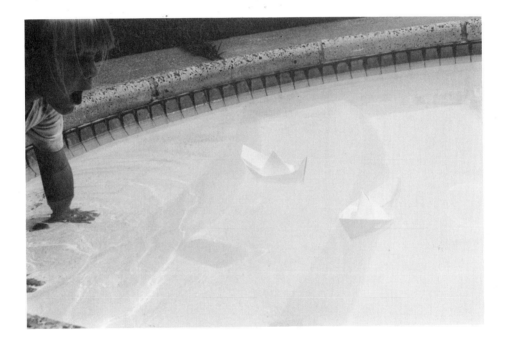

Following paper-folding directions requires spatial organization, concentration, and precision and offers opportunities for choice and decision-making in terms of colors and objects selected. Paper folding is ordinarily a bilateral task and is one of the few activities that requires finger extension.

As with all tasks, be certain the object is viewed by the client as age appropriate. Although paper folding appeals to children and adults alike, the projects described here are more suitable for children and are easier to make than origami because of their larger size. However, adults like to make them for and with children. Traditional origami, which is more complex and is on a smaller scale, can be done by older children and adults. Instructions for origami are found in packages of origami paper, as well as at bookstores and libraries.

Printing

Printing allows the production of multiple copies of a single design. Simple methods of printing were forerunners of the mechanized printing used in industry.

These activities are useful for developing shape recognition and other aspects of perceptual acuity.

Block Printing

The linoleum block is a derivation of the wood block used for printing in earlier times. Block printing can be done on individual sheets, or the block can be locked up in a chase and used to print multiple copies on a press. Block printing is used commercially for the production of valuable limited-edition prints.

You will need:

Linoleum block
Chisel
Brayer
Ink

1. Prepare your design. *The design on the block will be the reverse of the printed design.* Be particularly careful if you are incorporating letters or numbers into the design.

2. Darken the outline of the design with a soft pencil.

3. Trace the design onto the block by rubbing on the back side of the paper with a tooler or spoon. Remove the paper.

4. Use a chisel to remove the linoleum from the background or unprinted areas.

5. Ink the block with a brayer.

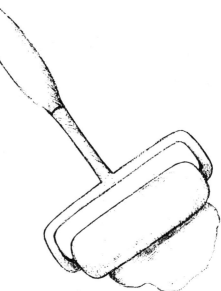

6. Turn the block onto the paper, and hammer it with a mallet, or put paper on the block and rub with a spoon.

7. Reink the block between printings.

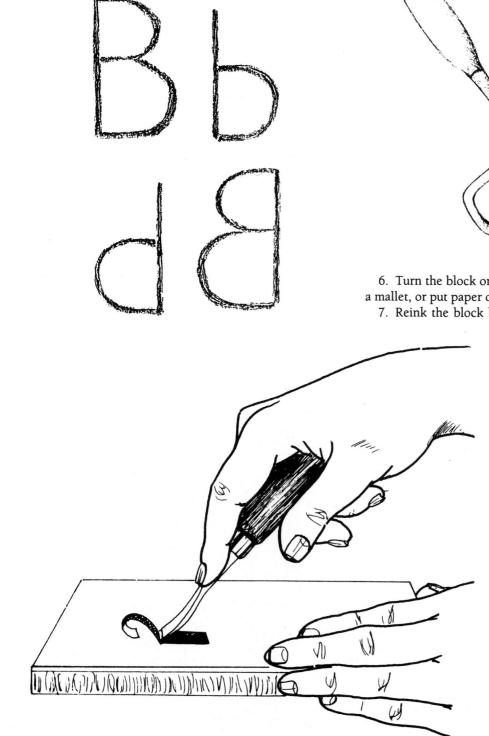

Adapted from Craft Techniques in Occupational Therapy. Department of the Army, Washington, DC, 1980, p 14-36.

Vegetable and Gadget Printing

Many simple methods of printmaking are interesting and inexpensive clinical activities. Some are very appealing to children yet can also be of interest to adults. These activities offer fun ways to decorate wrapping paper for gifts.

Printing blocks and plates can be made of many things:

1. Carve a raised design into a potato. Dip the potato into a sponge saturated with water paints and then press the potato onto paper. Cut vegetables such as cabbage and okra also can be used.
2. Items such as spools, sink suction gadgets, bottle tops, cloth, cardboard, and leaves also can be used.
3. Draw designs onto styrofoam grocery trays with a pencil.
4. Squeeze polymer glue onto cardboard and allow it to dry raised.
5. Draw a design onto corrugated cardboard. Cut away the excess, exposing the fluting.
6. Run an inked brayer onto the plate and print just as with a block print.

Stenciling

Stenciling is a good method of personalizing stationery. Purchase an inexpensive package of blank paper and envelopes, imprint them, and repack them in the box for a gift. Stencils can also be used to decorate furniture and walls.

You will need:

Stencil paper, acetate, or used x-ray film
Stencil brush—a round cluster of firm bristles, flat at the end
X-Acto knife
Package of stationery or other blank paper
Tempera paints
Masking tape

1. Choose or design a simple silhouette pattern. Trace it onto acetate or x-ray film. Do not use cardboard because it is too porous.
2. Cut the design out of the acetate with a sharp craft knife.
3. Secure the stencil to the paper with masking tape to prevent it from being dislodged as you work.
4. Dip the flat end of the stencil brush into the paint. Remove the excess by rubbing the brush lightly on a paper towel.
5. Hold the brush flat against the paper, starting around the edges of the stencil. Apply the paint in a circular motion, continuing into the center of the design until the area is evenly colored. Another simple way to stencil is to apply color to a sponge and dab until the area is completely filled.

Several stencils can be combined to create a more complex design (Fig. 7–17). For multicolor designs, print all items of a given color before changing stencils. Do the lightest colors first, then each subsequently darker tone.

Silk screening, like stenciling, creates multiple copies of the same design. Silk-screen frames can be purchased

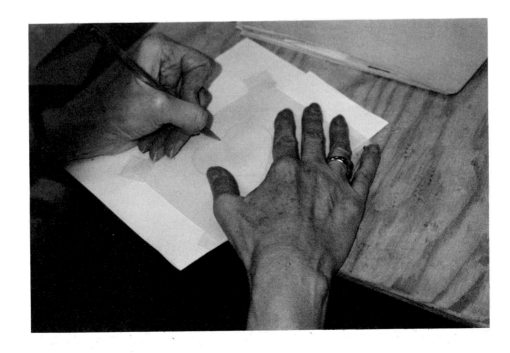

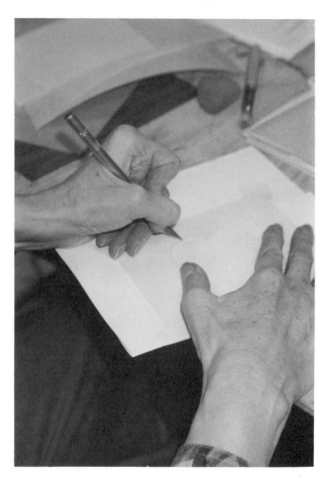

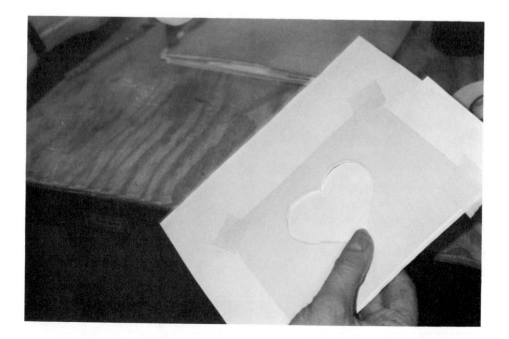

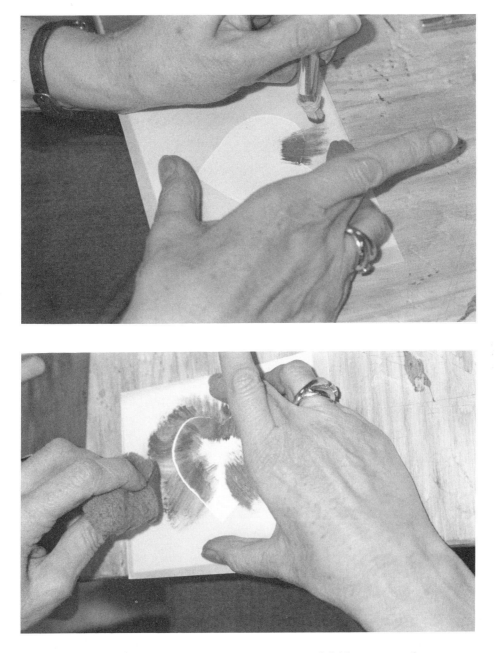

from a craft supplier. The frame is used to keep the stencil in place, and ink or paint is formed through the screen with a squeegee. A simple method of silk screening is to use water-soluble glue instead of a stencil to block the ink from passing through the screen. The glue can be removed from the screen by running it under warm water. A more sophisticated form of silk-screening is used by commercial printers to produce fine-quality prints.

Bookbinding

Mechanized printing ultimately led to the mass production of books and other reading materials. A creative method of folding press sheets into groups of pages, called signatures, made the production of books efficient and more readily available to the public. This marked advance in the production of written materials allowed ordinary people to obtain education, a right formerly available only to privileged individuals. These advances enabled society to change in many ways as it became possible to share information freely.

Early bookbinding used a combination of mechanical and hand tools (Figs. 7–18 and 7–19). Hand bookbinding has largely become a specialized art because machines do a more efficient job for large-scale manufacturing. The artisan's skill at this work remains valued in special places such as museums and libraries, and this craft has been kept alive for its ornamental qualities.

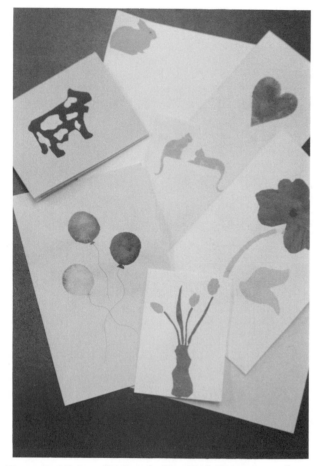

Figure 7–17. Stencil prints, by New York University students.

You will need:

White paper
Ornamental paper for inside cover
Awl
Clamps
Wooden press
Tapestry needle
Button thread
Beeswax
White glue
Cardboard
Fabric
Spoon
Spine cloth (organdy)

1. A signature is made from a single, folded sheet of paper. The number of signatures dictates the size of the book. An 11 × 17 inch sheet makes 16 pages at 4¼ × 5½ inches. Prepare enough signatures to make the size book you desire. Fold each signature according to the accompanying illustration.

2. Crease the edges of the signatures sharply with the edge of a spoon. Carefully slit the pages open with a letter opener. The torn edges distinguish the book as handmade, but the edges can be trimmed evenly with a guillotine paper cutter, if you prefer.

3. Pierce the spine edge of the signatures at 1-inch intervals.

4. Stitch the signatures together. Knot the thread.

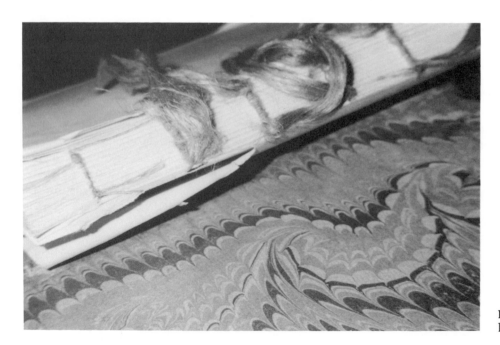

Figure 7–18. Bookbinding, Williamsburg, VA.

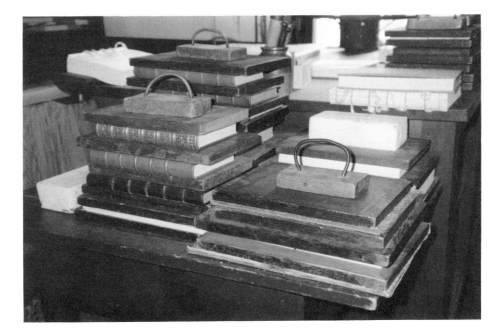

Figure 7–19. Bookbinding, Williamsburg, VA.

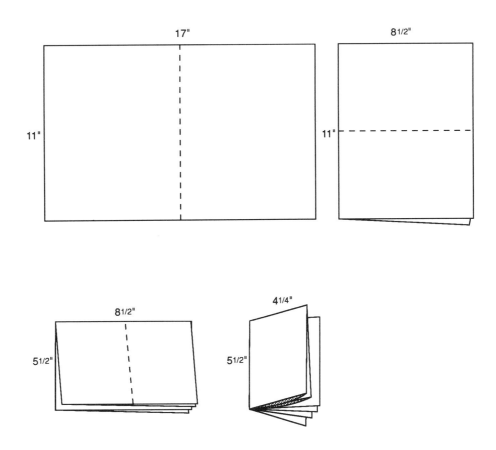

Starting with the last signature, go in and out of each hole through the creases, reversing direction in the next signature, and so forth. Reinforce the threads each time you tie to a new signature.

5. Clamp the signatures together in a wooden press, being sure the edges are even on all sides. The signatures should protrude ³⁄₁₆ inch from the press. Hammer the edges flat along the whole spine.

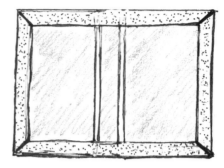

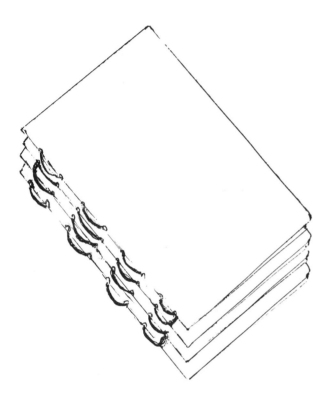

6. Glue a strip of cloth 2 inches shorter than the length of the spine and 4 inches wider than the width of the spine, centering it on the spine.

7. Cut 2 pieces of cardboard ½ inch longer and wider than the signatures and 1 piece the length and width of the spine. These form the covers and spine of the book.

8. Cut a piece of fabric double the width of the cardboards plus the spine, plus 2 inches. This will be the book cover.

9. Glue the cardboard covers to the fabric exactly ¹⁄₁₆ inch from the spine edge, centered top and bottom. Center the spine board on the fabric and glue it in place.

10. Fold the fabric over the covers. Miter the corners and glue the fabric down on the inside of the covers.

11. Glue the spine cloth to the front and back covers.

12. Cut 2 pieces of ornamental paper to fit the inside covers and first and last pages.

Creating one's own book can be a very rewarding experience. By using blank sheets, a truly personalized diary or album can be made. Limited editions of hand-bound printed work can be produced, but this consumes a great deal of time and requires a considerable degree of skill and patience. Bookbinding is an ideal activity for the individual who has extensive leisure time.

Photography

Photography was a natural progression from other two-dimensional reproduction techniques. Being readily able to reproduce the world as it appears, not as it is imagined, is a remarkable feat made possible by the camera. Photography's development from the simple box camera to today's instant and automatic cameras was made possible by sophisticated advances in chemical and other technologies. The ready adoption of photography into our modern culture was stimulated by the desire of people to record and share their experiences. Communication was expanded by the development of photography.

Photography is used for documentation as well as leisure pursuits. Since its development, it has been used to record the history of our time. Family events, wars, wildlife, and microscopic particles have all been recorded photographically.

Learning to take photographs can be as simple or complex as the photographer's interests and the applications for which the pictures are intended. The techniques described here apply to the 35-mm automatic camera only, because this book is for beginners. As with all techniques, as your interest is piqued, you may wish to expand your skills with input from other sources.

You will need:

Camera
Film
Batteries
Releases

GERI-REHAB, INC.
Occupational therapy
consultation
services

We are currently providing Occupational Therapy to you, your friend, or relative. In addition to providing therapeutic services, we are engaged in the study of occupational therapy rehabilitation techniques. We would appreciate the opportunity to film patient progress to aid us in providing improved treatment, developing research, and educating staff and other health professionals.

We request your signature below and thank you for your assistance in furthering our knowledge and advancing our rehabilitation skills.

Sincerely yours,

Estelle B. Breines, PhD, OTR, FAOTA
President

- -

Please read and sign the following:

I hereby authorize Geri-Rehab, Inc. to film the progress of
_____. I relinquish all rights to that film. The film is to be used for the study and the development of educational tools.

_____
Signature   Date

_____
Relationship

Courtesy of Geri-Rehab, Inc., Lebanon, NJ.

Before shooting any clinical pictures, be sure to obtain signed releases from patients and/or their guardians, particularly if you intend to use the pictures in publications or at educational seminars. Unless you have a release, you are violating people's rights to privacy.

Obtaining a Camera

Many families today have cameras in their homes, so you may already have access to one. If not, you may want to purchase one. Cameras range widely in price according to the number of features they have. Because cameras also can be rented, this may be a good way to make an educated decision about equipment choices. Also, you can always purchase a disposable camera.

Automatic cameras are close to foolproof for beginners. The term "automatic" describes the camera's ability to focus on the subject without it being set manually. No calculations are necessary. Adjustments for changes in lighting are made by the camera, not the photographer. Most automatic cameras will not operate if the shot is not well lit. The automatic camera takes much of the thinking out of photography.

Some automatic cameras also come with additional automatic features. These include lighting, loading, advancing, and rewinding the film. Be a prudent shopper and decide which features are important to you. Visit several camera shops and discuss your options before making your purchase.

Parts of the Camera

Lens. The eye of the camera. The lens opening, which is called an aperture, regulates the amount of light passing through the lens onto the film.

Viewfinder. An opening that enables the photographer to see what the camera sees.

Flash. Light source.

Shutter. Lever used to allow light to enter the lens and strike the film.

Film advance and rewind knobs. Film is threaded through rods attached to these knobs. Turning these knobs advances or rewinds the film. Some cameras advance the film automatically. Others need to be advanced manually.

Battery case. The motor and light require electricity to operate them. The batteries are the source of energy. Check them frequently. Batteries are as important as film. Without them the camera will not operate. Batteries left in the camera for an extended period of time can leak and damage it.

Selecting Film

SLIDES OR PRINTS. Slides are useful for presentations, but they require a projector or slide viewer to display them. Sometimes the cost of each and their developing differs. Prints are more useful for filing, mounting, and making reproductions in documents.

BLACK AND WHITE OR COLOR FILM. Black and white film is less costly than color film and makes better printed reproductions. On the other hand, most hobbyists prefer color prints because their lifelike appearance is more appealing.

FILM SPEED. Film is numbered according to its speed: for example, 100, 200, 400. The greater the number, the faster the speed of the film, and, generally, the higher the cost. For most amateur purposes, 100 speed, 35-mm print film is adequate. If you think the light on the subject may be insufficient, such as on a cloudy day, use a faster film such as 200. If your subjects will be moving, use 400. If you expect to have your prints published, use 400 film because it will offer greater resolution, and thus better reproductions.

Taking Pictures

DESIGN. To take good quality photographs, pay attention to design. The balance of contrasting colors, shapes, and subjects contributes to the design. View the scene as the camera sees it. In planning your shot, place an imaginary frame around the subject, just as the viewfinder does. Some practice with the camera will give you a better appreciation of how closely the viewfinder predicts the pictures you actually get. Examining your photos will allow you to make adjustments in your shooting.

DISTANCE. Distance from the subject is an important factor in getting good pictures. Many automatic cameras are limited in their ability to do close-up shots. On the other hand, new photographers often do not come close enough to their subjects. Practice taking shots from different distances.

FOCUS. Automatic cameras present some interesting focusing problems. They focus on the central and foremost item in the viewing field. Therefore, items of interest may be out of focus. For example, if a fence surrounds animals at the zoo, the camera may focus on the fence, and not on the animals! Take care not to focus on any item the camera sees that the eye tends to ignore.

LIGHTING. The light source should be coming from behind you. Do not face the camera into the sun or with the light coming from behind the subject. Sharp contrasts and very white subjects can fool the automatic camera into making false adjustments. Automatic cameras will not work if the lighting is inadequate. They usually will alert you to use a flash. Some flashes need to be set; others work automatically. Know your camera's capabilities before shooting.

SUBJECTS. If the subject of a photo is very important to you, take more than one shot of it, preferably from different angles. The cost of duplicating shots is negligible when compared with the possibility of having lost the opportunity to retake the picture.

DEVELOPING. Some photographers enjoy developing film because it allows them creative liberties, but the average person takes film to a professional for developing. Modern advances in technology have made developing services readily available virtually everywhere, even 1-day developing. Many developers offer duplicate prints for little additional cost.

Clinical uses of photography straddle the realms of therapeutic activity and documentation. Taking photographs can become an all-consuming hobby and lends itself to individual and group activity. Special photographs make welcome gifts.

Aside from using photography as a creative tool, the well-equipped clinic should always contain a camera for documenting clinical events. Nothing is more graphic than before and after photos illustrating change. Keep one camera loaded with slide film and one with print film to be ready for that shot that should not be missed.

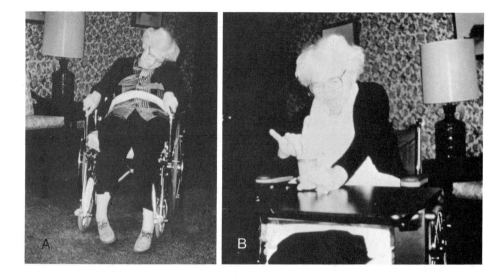

Courtesy of Geri-Rehab, Inc.,
Lebanon, NJ.

Videotaping*

Electronic transmission of images was a natural progression from the era of stills and moving pictures. When film was the primary means of preserving a moving image, the equipment was bulky and fairly difficult to use, and the cost of cameras, lights, and other necessary tools was prohibitive for all but the most serious filmmakers. Film also does not allow for instant viewing; it must be removed from the camera and then sent to a lab for processing. The invention of television and the subsequent widespread use of videotape ushered in an era of instant visual communication and offered many new advantages.

As equipment became smaller and more inexpensive, the use of video increased. Hand-held cameras were within the range of many people's pockets. Cameras, recorders, and editing devices found their way into homes, businesses, schools, and hospitals.

> Videotaping is a good tool for the clinic, whether for creative or other therapeutic purposes. Videotape includes sound, is reuseable, can be easily duplicated, and provides for immediate viewing. Video technology offers extraordinary opportunities for skill building. Making a videotape can be an excellent group activity during which clients can be encouraged to express themselves in a variety of ways.

The viewing of videos can be equally valuable. Social interactions can be taped and used both as evaluative and self-evaluative tools. The taping of soap operas, "drunk tanks" where alcoholics recover, and training and interviewing techniques, have all been used successfully as therapeutic tools. Training tapes are used to demonstrate techniques that are more readily understood by viewing them. Creative processes can be observed and analyzed. Clinical reasoning can be monitored. Clients can participate in and view scenarios involving family interactions, job interviewing, behavior modeling, or amateur news programs.

The therapist's repertoire is expanded by the video camera and videocassette recorder (VCR), which serve as both clinical and educational tools. Learning to make tapes allows the therapist to use this skill for documentation and clinical education and for guiding patients in use of the video camera as a creative tool for expression.

You will need:

Videocamera
Videorecorder
Editing equipment (optional)
Lighting
Videotapes
Television set
Tripod (optional)

All equipment must be compatible. Check specifications of tapes and equipment.

*Technical production information for this section was contributed by Mitchell Ehrlich, OTS.

Equipment Formats

A number of different kinds of equipment formats are available, despite the consolidation attempts of the major video hardware manufacturers. Primarily, they include ½-inch VHS, the older Betamax (Beta), and the newer Hi-8, or 8-mm, format. Keep in mind that these formats are not interchangeable. If you record in ½-inch VHS, you must play back that tape on a VHS machine. A ½-inch VHS camera-recorder combination is recommended.

Production Techniques

In most instances, the type of production done in a clinical setting is single-camera production, where one camera is used to do all the recording. Familiarize yourself with the camera by reviewing the instruction manual. If possible, consult with a video professional. Many hospitals have professional video departments that can provide consultation, and the source of purchase can often provide valuable advice.

In the clinic, most of your recording will be done "hand-held." Remember to hold the camera steady and avoid tilting or jarring the camera. For additional support, you can lean against a wall or rest on a table to reduce the amount of vibration and movement of the camera. Holding your arms close to your body helps eliminate camera movement. You may find a tripod useful.

Use the zoom control sparingly. The zoom will help you get closer to whatever you are shooting, but its use can be distracting. When using the zoom, use a slow, methodical movement.

Panning is moving the camera left or right. One of the most distracting techniques is panning rapidly. Move the camera slowly to allow the viewer to orient to what you are trying to show.

Most cameras today record very well under normal lighting conditions. If additional lighting is necessary, normal household lamps will do. You can also "bounce" light by using larger, white showcards to redirect sunlight or artificial light. Remember not to point the camera directly at a light source; extreme brightness can damage the camera.

Sound recording can pose a problem, depending on the environment. Usually, a microphone is mounted directly on top of the camera, pointed in the same direction as the lens. These microphones are omnidirectional; they are designed to record in a wide pattern. Try to limit extraneous noise in the environment if possible. Consider purchasing a hand-held unidirectional microphone that plugs into an auxiliary jack on the camera. This will allow you to point the microphone exactly where you want and will eliminate some of the ambient noise in the environment, such as street noises. Another alternative is to tape without sound and dub sound in later, either using music or dialogue.

Preparing Titles

Many higher-end cameras have the ability to do titles in the camera, but the controls for this option are often very difficult to figure out. Try large bold block letters, preferably black on a white showcard. Magnetic letters work well, as do felt letters. Sometimes other techniques can be effective, when they are suitable to the topic being shot. For example, colorful crayon drawings and lettering can be used to illustrate a video about children. Or, if you are shooting in the Occupational Therapy department, use the sign outside the department.

One word of advice. When recording your titles, shoot enough footage to allow the viewer to read the title, but not so much that the viewer is bored. A rule of thumb is to read the title yourself twice through the viewfinder when recording.

Telling the Story

A certain amount of "preproduction" planning must be done before you begin shooting your videotape. Think of what you want to accomplish with the tape, who your audience is, where the video will be shot, and what problems you might encounter. Professionals employ a technique called "storyboarding," in which each scene is actually drawn on a piece of paper to visualize how the shots will look.

When you are ready, write the script. Include descriptions of scenes and dialogue, if appropriate. For each scene, note needed props or special effects. Distribute scripts to everyone in the crew. During a meeting of the crew, each member should mark his or her copy of the script to indicate special responsibilities.

Because you are shooting with one camera, you need to use a technique called "editing in the camera." This refers to planning ahead to shoot the story in the exact sequence in which it will appear. So, if you want a title in the beginning of the program, you need to shoot it first. If you forget, it will be difficult to add it later.

Use the rule of long shot, medium shot, and close-up shot in your production. A long shot is an establishing shot; it orients viewers to the environment and lets them know where they are. A medium shot moves the viewer closer to the action. A close-up brings the viewer into the action. Close-ups of hands and faces are very effective. Remember to hold the camera very still when shooting a close-up, because motion tends to be exaggerated when close. A tripod may be helpful.

Whenever appropriate, humor is a valuable tool. When humor is used, the audience is more likely to pay attention to the message and to remember it. However, be cautious. Not everyone has the same standards for humor. Know your audience and your topic.

Assigning Roles

Depending on the extent of the production, the following division of labor may be helpful in assigning tasks.

Producing. The producer generally conceives of the project, structures the financing, obtains permissions, arranges for site use, and supervises the job through to its completion and distribution.

Writing. The writer may conceive an idea or write the script based on a submitted idea.

Directing. The director guides the shooting, keeping overall control of the various elements that contribute to the completion of the shoot, such as sequencing, acting, and environmental and technical elements.

Acting. Actors act out the script as directed.

Props. The prop master procures items, sometimes including environments to enhance the story line with visual support.

Costumes. The costumer procures and sees to the care of clothing to support the story line.

Camera. The camera operator shoots the story under direction.

Lighting. The lighting engineer provides sufficient lighting for scenes.

Editing. The editor splices and deletes scenes under direction.

Duplicating. The processor reproduces sufficient copies of completed works for distribution purposes.

One individual can do it all, or the job can be divided among several people.

CASE EXAMPLES

Alice C. is a 15-year-old high school sophomore from a very religious family. She recently showed signs of depression resulting in a suicide attempt. Her family reports that she had a relationship with a boyfriend of whom they disapproved, and they refused to let her participate in extracurricular activities. She began to spend long periods of time locked in her room, emerging at odd hours for meals. After the suicide attempt, she was admitted to the acute psychiatric ward at a local hospital and from there was transferred to a private facility for disturbed adolescents.

GOALS

1. Heighten feelings of self-efficacy.
2. Reestablish peer relationships.
3. Provide opportunities for creative expression and insight, using creative projects as projective techniques.
4. Encourage communication with parents.

ACTIVITIES
Reading, bookmaking, stenciling.

Initially, Alice resisted "talk therapy" sessions, attempting to repeat her pattern of isolation. The occupational therapist discovered that Alice liked to read and provided her with books in order to develop rapport. At one point, she urged Alice to try to make a book and showed her how to do it. Alice covered the book with a stencil design of her own. Alice was encouraged to use her book as a means of communication, first with herself, then with her therapists and psychiatrist. Because she had a flair for design, she was encouraged to make some cards and send them to friends in hopes of reestablishing relationships with her peers. Alice and her parents began to attend family therapy sessions. While Alice showed them how book signatures are made, they explored their relationships with one another.

R.J., 15; E.B., 17; L.M., 14; and J.O., 16; are adolescent single mothers, all with a history of drug abuse. They attend a special school where they can complete their high school education and learn to care for their babies. The goals of the program are to educate these youngsters so they remain drug free and acquire experiences and skills that can be used in the workplace. Specific goals for these young mothers are to:

1. Improve self-image and confidence.
2. Develop child-care skills.
3. Develop work and self-care skills.

ACTIVITY
Prepare videotapes to use as training tapes for others in similar circumstances.

These girls came from impoverished homes and had little exposure to costly videotaping equipment. The program encourages the use of modern equipment to fill in cultural gaps in their learning, to prepare them for experiences in the work world. Consequently, the group decided to prepare videotapes to use as training tapes for other students. They selected topics, wrote scripts, prepared graphics outlining the techniques, and assigned roles for production of the tape. Using their babies as models, each member of the group demonstrated a child-care technique for the camera. They offered each other constructive suggestions to improve their appearance for their camera debut. They prepared for the videotaping by practicing the skills they later demonstrated. They each learned to operate the camera and the VCR. The girls showed the tapes at an assembly program at the end of the semester and received a commendation from the principal.

ELECTRIC WIRING

Times and Events

Virtually no modern equipment, household or industrial, can operate without electricity. Electricity is the energy source of our modern civilization. Wire is used for the conduction of electricity for untold industrial purposes. Copper, a good conductor of electricity, is encased in a protective sleeve of rubber or other nonconducting material to form wire. Electric wire is sold in rolls or by the yard. It is manufactured according to Underwriter Laboratory (UL) codes, which dictate the purposes and specifications for each kind of wire. Whenever you work with electricity, be certain to use the correct wire and to check that the covering of the wire is intact.

Although we are apt to take electricity and the use of wire for granted, an awareness of how it works is helpful in knowing how electric items are adapted for special uses. One way to learn about electricity is to wire a lamp. In the process, you will develop confidence in your ability to handle electricity safely.

The construction, adaptation, maintenance, and repair of electric equipment for special rehabilitation needs is within the scope of occupational therapy practice. Therefore, becoming adept at these skills prepares one for building competency in basic aspects of rehabilitation technology. Developing skill in wiring can be the first step in learning how to adapt electrically operated equipment to meet patients' special needs. Even when the need for adaptations exceeds your own skills, some knowledge in this area will help you to collaborate with others in the design of rehabilitation equipment.

Caution: Electricity can be dangerous. When working with electric circuitry, turn off and unplug the item. Sometimes the power to an outlet must also be turned off.

Wiring a Lamp

Lamps can be made of many objects and materials, but they must be wired properly to operate (Fig. 7–20). Electricity from a central source is transmitted through a plug, along an electric wire, to a socket into which a light bulb is inserted. To work, the electric circuit that is formed in this process must be intact.

You will need:

Lamp base (see Woodworking section, page 156)
Threaded metal tube
Bolt
Electric wire
Plug
Lamp socket
Bulb
Wire stripper

1. Insert a threaded metal tube through the hole at the top of the lamp. Bolt in place.
2. Insert a 12-foot piece of electric wire through the metal tube, leading out the base of the lamp.
3. Separate one end of the wire into 2 sections and tie. Use for the lamp socket.
4. At each end of the wire, strip off the rubber coating for 1½ inches, uncovering 2 separate copper wires.
5. Wire one end of the wire to the lamp socket and one end to the plug. Carefully wrap each wire around a screw, being certain that the wires do not touch each other. Tighten the screws securely so the wires do not slip.

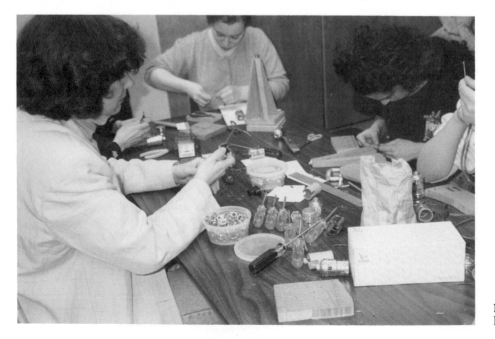

Figure 7–20. Students wiring lamps.

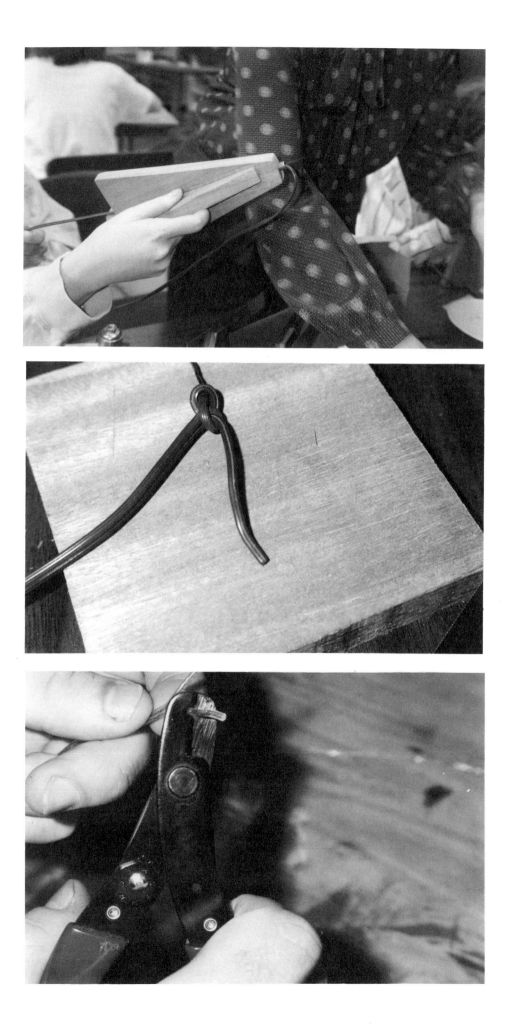

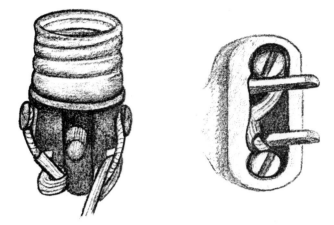

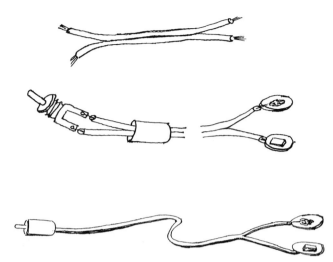

6. Replace the cover over the prongs of the plug.

7. Place a bulb in the socket. Plug in the lamp and turn on the switch. If you have wired the lamp correctly, it will light.

8. Attach a lampshade with a harp, or clip the shade to the bulb.

Penny Switches

A simple switch used to operate various items is a penny or single-contact switch. Copper pennies are used because they are good conductors of electricity.

You will need:

2 copper pennies
Adhesive-backed foam sheeting (½ × ½ inch, ⅛ inch thick)
Steel wool
Wire
Single socket plug (jack)
Soldering iron
Solder
Flux

1. Cut a 12-inch length of wire.

2. Separate one end of the wire into 2 separate wires. Strip the coating 1 inch from each end, exposing the wires.

3. Polish the pennies with steel wool.

4. Solder a penny to each of the wires, as follows: Heat the soldering iron. Apply flux to 1 of the pennies. Lay the wire against the penny. Hold the solder 1 to 2 inches above the wire. Heat the solder with the soldering iron.

5. Solder the 2nd wire and penny. Allow the metal to cool. Tug the wire to test its adherence to the copper. If the wire comes loose, resolder.

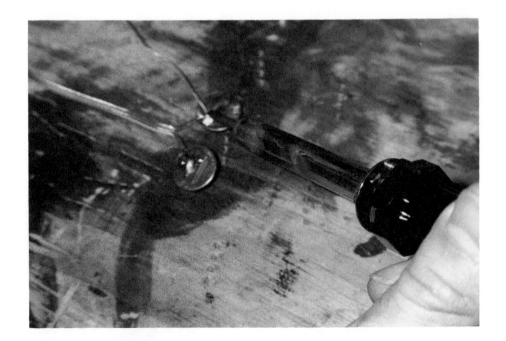

6. Cut out a small square of foam material and secure it between both pennies as shown. The foam keeps the pennies from making contact and completing the circuit until you want it to.

7. Cover the pennies with electric tape.

8. On the other end of the wire, separate into 2 separate wires. Wire the jack to the wires. Solder each wire to the screw.

9. Insert the jack into the socket of a battery-operated radio, tape player, or toy. Turn on the equipment to activate the battery. Touching the pennies together will complete the circuit, causing the item to operate.

> Hot solder runs in an instant, so it requires speed and dexterity to remove it quickly. The soldering iron and hot solder can cause burns. Work on a heat-proof surface, undisturbed.

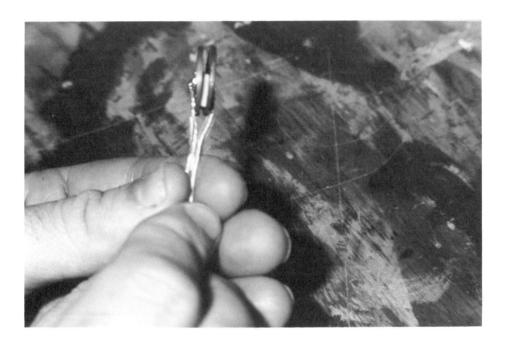

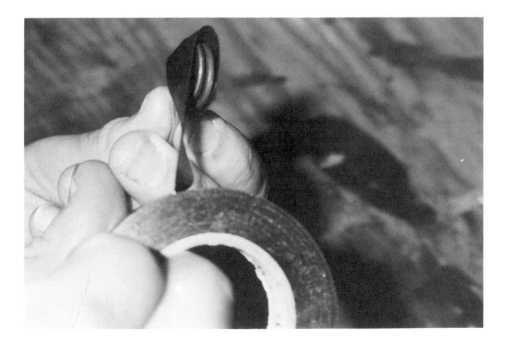

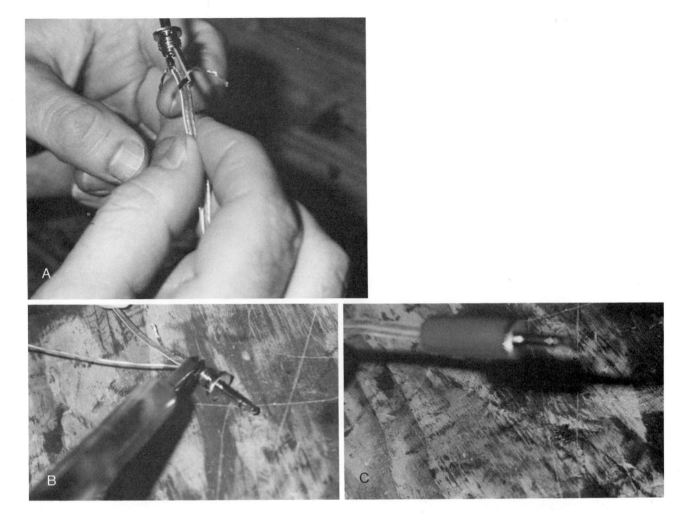

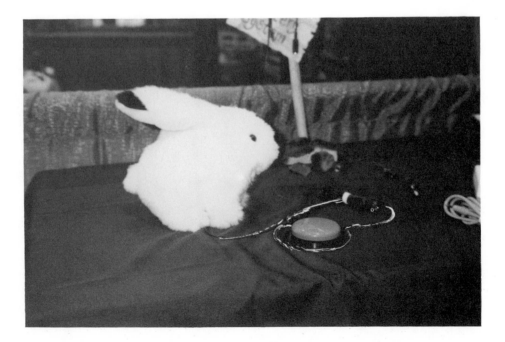

Adapting a Toy

Components are available from electronics and rehabilitation suppliers to adapt toys and other equipment. Such items are fitted with customized switches that allow children with limited strength and other capabilities to operate them.

Battery adapters and specially adapted switches are used to adapt toys. A battery adapter is a circuit interrupter fitted with a jack. The male jack is inserted into a female socket in a specialized switch to complete a circuit. Jack and receptacle must be the same sizes. Standard sizes are available, but some items may not be available in compatible sizes. If the jack is incorrect for the switch you wish to use and a correct one is not commercially available, rewire with a jack that fits correctly.

1. Insert the flat end of the battery adapter between the battery and the contact.
2. Plug the battery adapter jack into the adapted switch.
3. Turn on the equipment.
4. Operate the adapted switch to complete the circuit.

> This kind of switch will activate transistor radios, tape players, toys, and other such electric devices with a touch, a useful skill for an individual with limited abilities. A radio or tape recorder can be adapted to either turn on or off when the circuit is completed, allowing the therapist to select the most valuable stimulus for a particular patient and to modify it when necessary. The same adaptation can be inserted into a variety of toys, keeping the child's interest stimulated.

> Learning to wire electronic equipment helps one to understand its operation. It also helps one to be alert to costs. If you consider the cost of a therapist's time, the cost of preparation often exceeds the cost of purchasing finished equipment. A good rule to follow is: buy first, manufacture second. Make equipment only if items are not commercially available, or if you can produce them more inexpensively, considering all costs. This is a good rule to follow for all adapted equipment.

Circuitry

Circuit boards are complex wiring systems that can direct electric charges selectively. Wired circuit boards used to play a significant role in the manufacturing of electronic equipment. They are no longer used in industry because of the remarkable advances in miniaturized circuitry made possible by silicon chips. Computers are modern advances on circuit boards. The computer's silicon microchips are substituted for wiring, enabling incredible miniaturization and speed.

> Circuitry boards can sometimes be found in hobby shops and may be of interest to you or your patients. Constructing these can be popular leisure time activities and can be used to test and improve concentration, accuracy, dexterity, and other work-related skills.
>
> Complex wiring systems are used in model railroads, a popular leisure activity (Fig. 7–21).

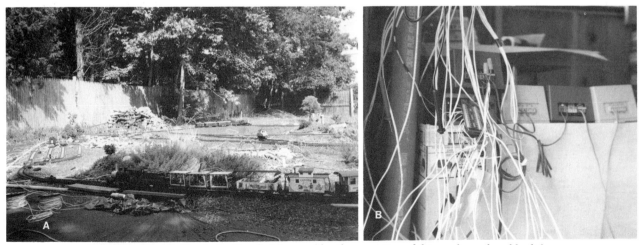

Figure 7–21. (*A*) Nearly 1 mile of wiring enables the operation of this garden railroad built by a retired executive. (*B*) Model railroad control center.

CASE EXAMPLE

Billy R. was an adopted, nonambulatory, nonverbal male with a chronologic age of 7 but a developmental age of 18 months. He was diagnosed with fetal alcohol syndrome, exhibiting symptoms of severe hypotonia, deficits in visual tracking, and limited attention span, resulting in the lack of play skills. Billy attends a day training school and lives at home with his parents and siblings who, while attentive, often are at a loss as to how to engage Billy in activity.

GOALS

1. Increase attention span.
2. Increase tracking ability.
3. Develop awareness of cause and effect.

ACTIVITY

Billy was encouraged to move a toy car adapted with a single-switch device activated by a pressure pad, by pressing on the pad with his hand. Different movable toys which had noises and lights were used to vary the activity and stimulate his interest and attention. These activities heightened his awareness of his own ability to cause change in his environment. Billy's parents and siblings were instructed in these activities, and the family bought several adapted toys for Billy for his birthday. The parents were also advised to install a touch switch at the base of a lamp in Billy's room to give him some control over his environment as he develops.

COMPUTERS

Times and Events

Computers have become part of everyone's lives in a remarkably short period. Banks, telephone systems, schools, grocery stores, and industries rely on computers to ever-increasing degrees, and they are gaining wider and wider usage throughout the world.

Computers are available in a number of forms. Mainframe computers are large internal networks. Personal computers are desktop models. Some portables, called laptops, are as small as a notebook; and even smaller, handheld notepads are available on the market.

Despite their differences, some aspects of computers are universal, so learning one operating system can make it easier to learn to operate another. On the other hand, the habits developed in using one system often make people resistant to changing to other systems.

Selection of a computer should be made with in-depth research and expert advice. The primary focus should be on the application software available to satisfy the user's needs. The secondary consideration should be the best hardware to run the chosen software. The tertiary focus

should be on the technical support available for both hardware and software to help solve the problems you will inevitably face.

The public's use of computers in everyday living validates the use of computers clinically, for the tools of everyday living are of necessity the tools of occupational therapy. Consequently, whether operating as therapist or manager, the modern clinician can no longer function optimally without computer literacy.

Because advances in computer technology are evolving so rapidly and because at this point in time computers and programs made by different manufacturers are not entirely compatible, this section focuses only on the broadest applications of computers. Home and office computers are the focus here because they are most commonly encountered in clinical situations.

Skill in the use of a computer is gained, as are all skills, through practice and mastery. As with all skills, computer skills cannot be learned by reading about them; they must be learned by doing. Therapists must gain computer fluency before they use the computer as a tool to meet individual patient needs.

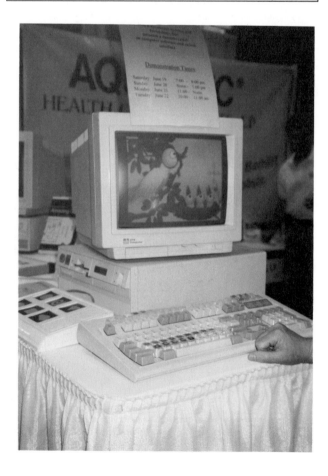

Specialized Terminology and Applications

The typical computer used in the clinic, home, or office includes a monitor, a keyboard, and perhaps a mouse or a track ball, a central processing unit, one or more disk drives and/or a hard drive, a printer, and sometimes a modem. Essentially, the operation of a computer depends on the interface between its hardware and software and the person using them. Learning computer jargon is the first step in learning its operation.

Hardware

Input Devices

Input devices are the means one uses to enter data into the computer. Input devices take several forms. Among these are the following:

Joystick. A handheld rod that moves 360 degrees or can be configured in quadrants to activate various controls. The joystick is customarily used to play games, but it can be adapted to other uses.

Keyboard. A display board that ordinarily contains 80 or more moveable keys. Most keyboards are modeled after the QWERTY design of the average typewriter. "QWERTY" is named for the first six upper left-hand keys. Keyboards can be obtained in other configurations, such as DVORAK. Programs to reconfigure keyboards for special needs are also available. Computer keyboards also contain function keys and numeric pads that are used to trigger various commands and perform computations.

Mouse. A handheld device containing a ball that moves the cursor on the screen. When the cursor is on the desired location, a button is pressed to activate a command.

Track ball. Operates like a mouse, but the device is stationary with a ball set into it. The ball is turned by the palm or fingers.

Light pen. A handheld, light-operated rod that is touched directly to a screen to activate the computer.

Power pad. A flat surface device that translates pressure into electric surges, allowing a gridlike configuration to be used for various input purposes.

Puff-sip device. A strawlike device that switches on and off by using air pressure blown into or sucked out of a tube. This device has been adapted for quadraplegics to enhance their independence in travel, communication, and environmental control.

Cables. Specialized electric wiring; the plugs are specially configured to connect hardware units to one another. Cables allow peripheral devices such as keyboards and video screens to interface.

Input devices provide therapists with many options from which to select devices appropriate for accessing the computer to meet special needs. For example, someone who cannot operate a keyboard because of manual deficiencies may be able to use a single stroke device, a mouse, or a head wand or a mouthstick to accomplish the same task. Compatability of device, computer, software, and user must be sought, and assured by the manufacturer prior to purchasing equipment. Both high- and low-tech adaptations can be designed to operate computers.

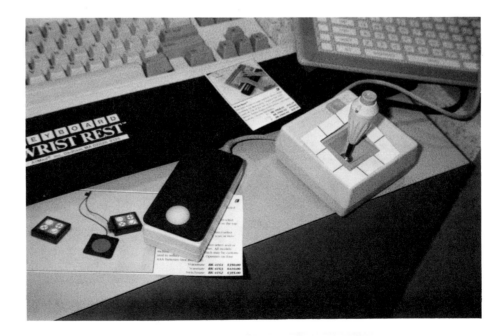

Central Processing Unit

The central processing unit (CPU) is the brain of the computer. It serves as the memory bank and processes information. Data are imported, sorted, and exported from here to the output devices.

CPUs are built on a binary system of bits and bytes. A bit is the smallest unit of the computer. Each bit is an off or on electric element, represented as 0 or 1, the absence or presence of a circuit. Bytes are composed of 8 bits. These 8 bits are configured so that each designated sequence of 0 and 1 represent a letter, numeral, or other symbol. For example, 01101100 and 00110101 represent different symbols. Bits and bytes are the building blocks of computer technology by which CPUs function and interface with programs.

The number of bytes defines the amount of random access memory (RAM) a computer has. RAM is a committed portion of memory allocated to operate the CPU system. The larger the memory, the more information the CPU can process. The amount of memory dictates which programs the CPU can handle and how many can be handled at once. As you work on a document, it is stored in RAM, which is only available when there is power to the computer. When the power is cut off, the data in RAM is lost. To be "remembered," data must be stored in random operating memory (ROM).

ROM is another kind of computer memory. ROM is stored information that can be brought into processing. ROM can be created using data storage devices as floppy disks, hard drives, laser disks, and tape cassettes. Unlike internal hard drives, disks and tapes can be stored external to the computer. This permits the user flexibility, enabling movement of data from one physical location to another. A virtually unlimited amount of data can be stored in a very small amount of space with the use of hard drives, disks, and tapes.

In an extraordinarily brief period of time, advances in technology have improved the capacity of computer memory to such an extent that one should not wait to purchase a system. Although whatever one purchases now is certain to be considered obsolete in very short order, the advances in hardware and software currently available will probably remain functional for a long period to come.

Output Devices

Output devices enable the user to deliver processed information from a computer system in various forms. This information can be auditory, visual, or even tactile, such as in a temperature control device. Output devices include video screens, printers, audio mechanisms such as speech synthesizers, and other devices such as robots. Computer systems can operate several output devices, concurrently or sequentially. Output devices are selected to meet the needs of the task or the individual.

Surge Protectors

Surge protectors are highly recommended to minimize the danger of losing data because of electric surges and brownouts. Uninterrupted power systems (UPS) are the best way to protect a system from being affected by electric problems. They take over like a battery back-up when an electric problem develops.

Software

Software is a set of instructions designed to accomplish a specific set of tasks. These instructions are stored in a variety of forms depending on the design of the hardware and software. These forms include floppy disks, hard drives, tape cassettes, and laser disks. The information on the software interfaces with the computer and directs what is to be done.

Software has been designed for work-related tasks as well as recreational activities. In addition to its applications in manufacturing, its calculation and writing capabilities can be used for learning modules, word processing, business management, scientific research, data processing and storage, and games.

Choosing Software

Commercial software is available from many sources at costs that range widely. Public domain software, also known as shareware, is available at little to no cost to the user. Software is selected according to the use to which it is to be put and its compatibility with the hardware being used.

Whenever possible, select "user-friendly" software. One user-friendly software uses "icons." Icons are pictures that make it easy to recognize commands without having to commit them to memory. Icon-driven software is user-friendly because the same commands operate all software produced by that manufacturer. Therefore, once the symbols are learned, they can be applied universally. Icon-driven software is usually operated with a mouse, reducing the need to input commands with the keyboard. Examples include Macintosh (MAC) and Windows by Microsoft.

Word Processing

Word processing is a tool for written communication. It generates copy and retrieves, reproduces, edits, transmits, and stores copy in numerous ways. It enables a markedly increased speed of processing, while reducing the space necessary for storing data. Errors can be corrected easily, allowing accurate copy to be generated with a minimum of effort. Examples include World Perfect, Multimate, Ami, and Windows Write.

> Word processing permits one to produce perfect hard copies (paper documents) by making corrections before printing. This feature can raise the self-concept of a learning-disabled child immeasurably. Moreover, with adaptations, profoundly disabled or isolated individuals can communicate with skill, equality, and independence, performing tasks otherwise impossible for them without this tool.

Desktop Publishing

Desktop publishing is a sophisticated advance on word processing. It allows the user to design attractive and readable documents. Desktop publishing software permits typeface to be enlarged, altered, and configured in various ways. It allows the editor to view the page in segments as well as in its entirety and to make changes easily and quickly. Desktop publishing has been used to generate documents of all sorts: forms, fliers, advertising copy, manuals, instructions, texts, and so on. Examples include Ventura and Page Maker.

Spreadsheet

A spreadsheet is a vertical and horizontal grid into which formulas and numeric values can be programmed. In addition to calculating numerical data, spreadsheets allow one to create column and margin headings to describe the data. Examples include Visi-calc; Lotus 1,2,3; Quantro; and Quatro Pro for Windows.

> The bookkeeping and record-keeping processes spreadsheets permit can be useful to patients as well as therapists. Clinical uses include attendance records, budgets, financial status reports, inventory, and research.

Data Processing

Data processing allows information to be entered, stored, and sorted according to predetermined parameters. Names, addresses, and special information can be sorted by alphabet, zip code, and other categories to produce records, labels, and so on. Examples include Q & A, DBase, and Access.

> Collecting data, analyzing it, and generating reports can be a management tool. Inputting data can be focused toward vocational preparation. All the software items listed above can be used as work-training tools for appropriate patients.

> Activity analysis should be used to determine the characteristics of various software packages and their suitability for training patients in specific skills.

Games

Many computer games are appealing and compelling. Game software is available from many commercial sources. Games are devised to hold the interests of children as well as adults. Examples include Solitaire, Reversi, Pac Man, Nintendo, and Atari.

> Game software can be used to develop particular skills associated with attention to stimulus, eye-hand coordination, speed, response time, accuracy, cooperation, competition, and so on. Games can integrate the functions of mind and body in activities that simulate real-life phenomena and can therefore be very intriguing to the participant.
>
> While games are potentially beneficial, they must be selected with care. Otherwise, they may not offer appropriate stimulation; may not be interesting, fun, or demanding; may be too complex, either perceptually or cognitively; or may lock the individual into a useless, obsessive activity. Selecting appropriate game software for individual clients requires the same skills of analysis used for other activities.

Instructional Software

Instructional software is used for education and skill training. Such software is available for all ages. Computer skills can contribute to learning from preschool on. Some examples of instructional software border on games, but they are included here for their educational value. Examples include Pelican Creative Writing Series; Professor DOS; FirstByte Designer Discovery Kit; Learning Company Spellbound!; Castle Creator; Broderbund Carmen Sandiego Series; MECC Oregon Trail; Hi-Tech Expressions Big Bird's Delivery; Ernie's Big Splash; Fisher Price School Bus; Designware Designosauris, Creature Creator; Spectrum HoloByte Tetris; and Spinnaker.

> Self-pacing and independence can be learned, along with content, by using such methods. Therapists and students also may use instructional software for their own learning.

Rehabilitation Software

Specially designed software for rehabilitation uses is available from merchants and vendors who specialize in

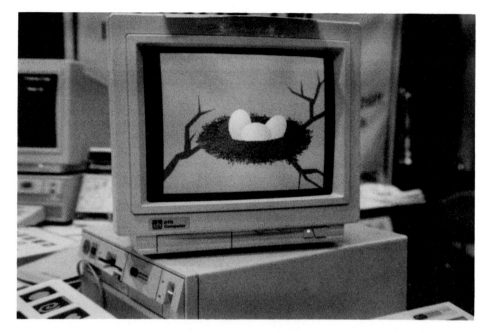

Figure 7–22. Display of software designed by Dr. Dina Loebl, OTR, Boston Education Systems and Technology (BEST), Inc., Boston, MA.

the development of these items (Fig. 7–22). See Commercial Sources of Supply in Appendix C for a list of software vendors.

Research

The computer is not only useful for research of all sorts, in this day and age its use is mandatory. Examples include SPSSx, Stat-pac, Ethnograph, Qualpro, Text Analysis Package, Textbase Alpha, Hyperqual, and OT Source.

> The computer is a valuable tool for data collection, recording, processing, and statistical and content analysis. Research software exists in the form of statistical packages, as well as software packages for ethnographic data analysis, bibliographic sorting, and library and data bank searches. Your clinic library should include software catalogs, and your local computer shop should be on your vendor and resource list.

Booting Up

Once you have your hardware and software, you are ready to "boot up." Booting is the start-up procedure that engages the software and hardware. Although computers vary, most follow these procedures.

If you have a hard drive, it must be loaded with the software you will be using. Instructions for loading software are found in the manuals that accompany each software package. Once the software is loaded, you can

begin to work. Because programs operate according to different commands, you must familiarize yourself with the manual that accompanies the software.

If you do not have a hard drive, insert the system's disk into the drive. Turn on the computer. Once the software has booted, remove the system's disk and insert the software on which you will be working.

Saving Data and Backing Up

Electronic equipment is vulnerable to electric surges, brownouts, or disconnections which can alter or erase data. Consequently, data should always be saved and backed up to prevent their loss.

Follow the directions shown in the manual for saving data. Data should be saved periodically as you work. Some people save data according to a timed period. Others take into account the critical nature of the material on which they are working. Save data more frequently when the weather is foul. It is best to discontinue working altogether when lightening threatens, to avoid electric outages and equipment damage. Whenever possible, program your computer to save automatically.

Backing up means making duplicate copies of data. Critical material should always be backed up on multiple disks or tapes. Computer buffs often back up data on disks identified as child, parent, and grandparent copies, marking their generations. Follow the directions in the manual for backing up. Backing up should be done daily or when changes have been made to documents. Backups of vital data should be stored in different locations for additional safety.

Viruses

The great advantage of carrying disks instead of reams of paper from place to place makes it easy and appealing to share information on disks. However, because of the risk of viruses, one needs to be very selective in bringing data from one computer to another. Viruses are computer messages that are imbedded in software, either deliberately or inadvertently, that cause information to be altered or deleted. Viruses are electronically transmitted from drive to drive when software is transferred from place to place.

Programs are available to debug software. Software should be checked regularly for viruses and other glitches, especially if disks and data are being shared. Examples include Norton Disk Doctor, Norton Anti-Virus, Central Point Anti-Virus, Virus Buster, and McAffee Scan.

Telecommunications

Telecommunications is a computer-based system interfacing software, telephone lines, and satellite communication systems. Electric impulses from one source are transmitted to a destination. Terms such as E-Mail, bulletin boards, data banks, BITNET, and local area networks (LANs) are the jargon of telecommunication. These tools are the means by which the modern world reduces distances between people so communication can occur.

Two commonly used telecommunication tools are the modem and the Fax.

MODEM. The modem translates a computer message into electronic signals. These signals are sent out on telephone lines to a distant location to be received by a source capable of reading the communication electronically. Documents are ordinarily transmitted using ASCII, a universally read computer language format. Through a modem, one can communicate on E-Mail, BITNET, CompuServe, Prodigy, and other such systems.

FAX. The Fax allows a written document to be read photoelectronically and instantly transmitted over telephone lines to a receiving Fax, which reverses the process. The electric impulses produce a "hard copy," or paper document, which is a facsimile, or Fax, of the original. Fax transmittal also can be made directly to and from computers equipped with FAX software. Here data are sent from screen to screen or can be scanned to send and be printed on receipt.

The uses of Fax have only begun to emerge. In addition to the standard office uses with which most people are familiar, Faxes are being used by children to share homework assignments, by office workers to order lunch, by builders to order construction materials, by homemakers to share recipes, and by toddlers to send drawings to their distant grandparents to keep as refrigerator art.

The ability to transmit information over great distances with a minimum of effort and unmatched speed is bound to be useful to populations with special needs. Telecommunications enable isolated or disabled individuals to meet on an even footing with people whose interests are allied with their own. It can enable them to be involved in the casual communication in which most people ordinarily engage, normalizing their socialization. Telecommunications can enable home-bound individuals, whatever the cause, to earn their living in an open market, to attend classes to broaden their education, and to communicate with friends with mutual interests in leisure pursuits.

Telecommunications are also used to expand educational opportunities from location to location. Clinics can use audio or video telecommunication systems to share information among therapists with similar clinical interests.

Adapted Equipment

Special adaptive equipment for the computer is readily available from a number of sources (see Commercial Sources of Supply in Appendix C for full addresses).

Keyboards (Angled, Hinged, and One-Handed Varieties)

DVORAK keyboard (first six upper left-hand keys) rather than standard QWERTY keyboard.

Kinesis Corp. of Bellevue, WA, has QWERTY keys set into two shallow wells, eliminates excessive reach for little fingers.

Anthony Hodges of Mountain View, CA, sells TONY!, a V-shaped board.

Health Care Keyboard Co., of Menomonee Falls, WI, makes a three-part QWERTY board, each part adjustable.

Voice-Activated Systems

Dragon Systems, Newton, MA, offers DragonDictate, DragonWriter, voice activated.

IBM Voice Type.

Kurzweil, Boston, MA, custom system.

Writing Systems

Free Software Foundation, Cambridge, MA. Cuts the number of keystrokes by completing commonly used words once the user hits the first three letters of the word.

Co-Writer (for Macintosh, piggybacks Mac Write), Don Johnston Co., Wauconda, IL.

Wrist Supports

Fox Bay Industries, Kent, WA.
North Coast Medical, San Jose, CA.
MicroComputer (Rubbermaid), Palo Alto, CA.
Silicon Sports, Palo Alto, CA.

CASE EXAMPLES

M.P., 68, is a retired executive. She developed degenerative osteoarthritis, which is localized to her spine, affecting her posture and mobility. M.P. lives alone in a co-op apartment on an adequate retirement income, but she feels isolated. She misses the socialization that work offered. A visiting therapist evaluated her situation and suggested the following:

GOALS

1. Increase opportunities for communication.
2. Develop leisure skills.
3. Develop feelings of self-efficacy.
4. Design and obtain a postural seating system to alleviate pain and reduce deformity.

ACTIVITY

M.P. was advised to enhance the computer skills she had begun developing on the job. A seating system was devised that allowed her to spend increased periods of time seated at the computer. M.P. learned to use a modem so she could communicate outside of her home. She instituted and coordinated a "newsletter of the air" (bulletin board) that permits communication among her former colleagues and other interested individuals. The newsletter deals with topics of general interest to the group, including job search opportunities and skills. She is busier now than ever and must remember to get up from her seat at regular intervals to move about.

The Future Is Now

To the being fully alive, the future is not ominous but a promise; it surrounds the present like a halo.

—JOHN DEWEY

Every activity described in this book is passé, obsolescent, or over the hill in one sense or another. As the ancient occupations of survival pass into the realm of the arts, new activities and tools emerge to take their place (Fig. 8–1). Nonetheless, each activity remains meaningful. Despite the changes history records, the media of former times retain their usefulness in the modern world. Our clothes are still made of cloth and leather, our furnishings of wood and metal, and, in many instances, the means used to make them are remarkably similar to those developed in the ancient past. Still, as history has recorded, the newest inventions are most exciting for each society, because these create the newest problems and thus the newest problems to be solved. These issues of time and change are as true for occupational therapists as they are for society at large.

THE MEANING OF ACTIVITIES

Meaningfulness governs our willingness to engage in activities. Patients can find meaning in activities designed in the past and in the present; some reach to the future for meaning and purpose in their lives. As therapists, we remain open to these perspectives, for they are fundamental to practice. Occupational therapy elicits performance; it acts with patients, not on them. It must remain sensitive to the needs and interests of patients in the world in which they live.

Knowing the evolution of an occupation allows the therapist to develop a sound therapeutic relationship because it helps the therapist understand the meaning of activity for the client. The patient-therapist collaboration depends on understanding the significance a given activity has for the patient as a functioning, or potentially functioning, member of society. Consequently, it is the therapist's obligation to remain alert to the meaning of activity for patients in a changing world.

ACTIVITIES CHANGE

Change continues at an ever-increasing pace, and its implications for society remain unpredictable. Who could have anticipated that the indispensable typewriter, which so markedly changed the nature of business procedures and social roles, would so rapidly become obsolete in this technologic age? Who would have thought that in a few short years, the mammoth and complex computer would be developed into a miniature toy for young children? The fantasy of rocket ships has become reality in just a few brief years. Buses can transport wheelchairs, not just people (Fig. 8–2).

Changes occur so swiftly in the modern era that one can no longer produce an object or a book that is "up to date." Given that situation, how can any therapist feel prepared? This question, as much as any other factor, underlies therapists' feelings of uncertainty and their lack of confidence. This sense of inadequacy must be reversed. Change is a condition that will never be resolved.

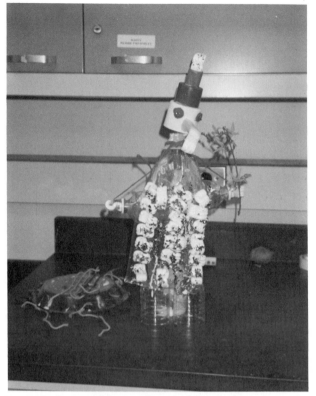

Figure 8-1. Assemblage sculpture of found plastic materials, by New York University occupational therapy students.

In fact, change is the essence of adaptation to which the profession is committed. Consequently, a positive perspective toward change must be adopted. Occupational therapists must recognize that their special philosophy is valuable in helping them to see potential and solution. Each new venture, each new patient, must be looked on as a new question, a quest for certainty. It is the therapist's job to devise creative solutions to resolve these uncertainties. Furthermore, when uncertainty is resolved, confidence builds for patient and therapist alike. Change is the future for which occupational therapists are prepared by their education and training. Finding solutions for new problems is met by the creativity for which occupational therapists are renowned.

THE ROLE OF THE THERAPIST

Each new invention with which society is presented is potentially a problem to be resolved in the clinical environment. The therapist's job is to use creativity fostered by knowledge to point the way to the solution of these problems. The therapist should be a role model for risk taking, thereby engendering confidence in the patient. Together, patient and therapist must collaborate in solving problems, using tools that are meaningful for the patient and, at the very least, are familiar to the therapist.

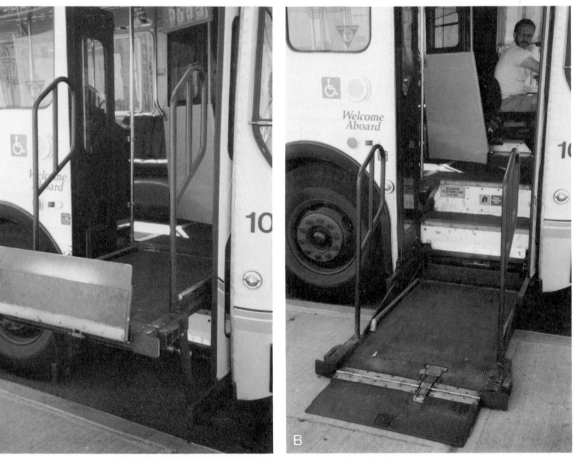

Figure 8-2. Bus accessibility mechanism, Seattle, WA.

Therapists must be prepared for practice not only with skills we know have been meaningful in the past but also with a reverence for uncertainty, because we can only imagine how the world and its tasks will change with time. Superconductors, monorails, and laser-driven computers are already with us; however, because their applications are still limited, they offer us only a peek into the future. Computers can be held in the hand, but our insights into their future applications are limited. The speed of travel and communication and the levels of automaticity these new opportunities will bring to human functioning can only be imagined at this point in time. As these new technologies become familiar tools, they will become absorbed into people's active lives and into children's preparation for living, while their implications for practice will emerge as well.

THE EFFECT OF CHANGE ON OCCUPATIONAL THERAPY

Occupational therapy was designed to respect and use the active occupations of the past, in order to understand their implications for human activity in the modern world, and beyond. Change was an expectation. Inherently, therapists always knew this. Throughout its history, the profession has moved along with the times, incorporating every new active occupation into practice as quickly as it was devised, while retaining the valuable skills of the past.[1] In the past, certain members of the profession have felt distressed as the field changed and grew, because there was little appreciation that the profession was designed for change, and that the new occupations were theirs as a birthright. Some reacted as if the old and the new were in conflict. Few recognized that occupational therapy derived its foundation from occupational genesis, whereby the end for human inventiveness is never in sight.

The world, as seen through the activities of its inhabitants, is in a constant state of becoming. Rabbi Emil Gustave Hirsch, founder of the first school of occupational therapy, professed: "Genesis is a divine poem whose last line has not yet been written."[2] In showing us that the world is constantly evolving through adaptation, he led us to understand that the future is not only open to change, but also that change is anticipated and welcome. Furthermore, in promulgating this belief in adaptation, occupational therapy was validated.

Adaptation is the profession's motto, evolution its theme. The basic tools of therapy—activity and its anal-
ysis, grading, and adaptation—can be applied without restriction to the promotion of development, learning, and health. These tools of practice enable the therapist to bring every new occupation into the clinic and to bring these occupations out of the clinic into the world at large.

Changes in therapeutic practice are taking place at the same rate of speed that the rest of society is experiencing. From the hospital environments of traditional practice, therapists have followed their patients back into their communities, as much to escape the narrow limitations of their own thinking, as to escape the restrictions of others. In doing so, therapists have learned that adaptation often can be applied best in the environments where activities ordinarily take place: the home, the school, and the workplace. Instead of simulating society, as Dewey did in the Laboratory School and as early therapists emulated in the hospitals and clinics, therapists of today have become a part of the community. They apply their skills in the real world by adapting activities to real-life patient problems. By taking their skills to the sites where the problems occur, therapists can better serve their patients—and by meeting patients' needs, the profession can be viewed in all its glory.

Following their instincts and their philosophy by applying the tools for change in the most sophisticated form, more occupational therapists are meeting the future with certainty and confidence, garnering the respect the profession deserves. Today's therapists should be confident that the profession was founded by great scholars and seers to meet the future in just this way. Therapists should recognize that the oldest and the newest tools of society are, and always will be, their own, by virtue of their heritage. Furthermore, therapists should understand that it is their obligation to keep pace with society's inventiveness and to meet their patient's needs for meaningful activity, whether those needs originate in the past, the present, or the future.

REFERENCES

1. Smith, RO, Hamel, J, Rein, J, et al: Technology as an occupational therapy treatment modality. OT Week, March 5, 1992.
2. Hirsch, EG: Laureate oration delivered at the commencement exercises of the Hebrew Union College, Friday evening, June 24, 1892. In Proceedings of the Union of American Hebrew Congregations 4:2951–2963, 1891–1897. American Jewish Archives, Cincinnati Campus, Hebrew Union College–Jewish Institute of Religion.

APPENDIX A

To the Faculty

This book is based on a two-semester sequence of activities courses designed by the author and offered at New York University's Department of Occupational Therapy since 1988.[1] These courses may interest you if you are designing or reorganizing your curriculum. Many more activities are described in this book than are offered in these classes. Select activities that fit your space and budget, that are appropriate to clinics in your region, and that you yourself enjoy. Schools that do not offer activities courses within the occupational therapy curriculum may wish to use this book to guide either home study or the selection of courses outside the occupational therapy program.

COURSE DESCRIPTIONS

Lectures cover the material outlined in this book and in *Origins and Adaptations: A Philosophy of Practice*. Laboratories follow the theme of occupational genesis, sequencing through the history of active occupation, and demonstrating the role of crafts as a therapeutic tool.

First Semester

The first semester begins with a workshop that introduces students to insights about the uniqueness of individuals as well as the power of groups, revealed through various activity experiences. Each week thereafter a different medium is taught and is accompanied by activity analysis. Two projects each of clay, basketry, and leather are offered to explore the concepts of grading and adaptation.

Laboratory activities follow this sequence:

Pinch pot
Coil pot
Wooden base basket
Reed basket
Leather case, personally designed, single cordovan
Leather case, prefabricated, double cordovan
Latch hooking
Macramé
Cardboard weaving
Machine-sewn stuffed doll (two partners work together on this project)

The semester ends with a trip to the American Museum of Natural History where students visit the halls of Northwest American Indians and South American peoples to compare the influence of environment on occupations in diverse cultures. On their return to the laboratory, students select a theme and clan leaders for a festival. They choose roles, decorate the environment, prepare food, and select and conduct activities in a "rite of passage."

Assignments

Logs are submitted for each medium (clay, reed, leather, fibers, fabric), in which students integrate concepts learned in lectures and readings with observations made in laboratories. All written assignments are word processed.

Each student teaches one other student an activity not taught in class. Activities vary from year to year according to students' interests. Students prepare teaching guides, including directions, costs, and sources, and distribute them to the class. Notebooks are kept of directions, samples, and so on.

Second Semester

The second semester focuses on characteristics of industrial and technologic work. Principles learned in the first semester are demonstrated using modern examples.

Laboratory activities follow this sequence:

Tissue paper greeting cards
Origami
Stenciling
Copper foil mold
Wire jewelry
Wooden lamp, wired
Penny switch soldering
Videotape presentations
Plastic crafts from found materials

Assignments

Students observe and compare "skilled" and "unskilled" work as a basis for discussing biases about work roles.

Each student visits a different work site; researches the industry; assesses work roles, the environment, safety, and health issues; and suggests adaptations. Reports to the class give students a wide overview of the breadth of work opportunities and demands.

Three activities are analyzed, including a newly learned computer program of each student's choice.

Small groups create videos on the topic of work and present them to the class.

REFERENCES

1. Breines, E: Media education based on the philosophy of pragmatism. Am J Occup Ther 43:461–464, 1989.
2. Breines, E: Origins and Adaptations: A Philosophy of Practice. Geri-Rehab, Lebanon, NJ, 1986.

APPENDIX B

Tools and Equipment for the Clinic

Every clinic must be outfitted with basic tools and materials appropriate to the clients it serves. A well-equipped clinic should have a broad variety of tools and materials. If cost is a concern, you will need to make choices. Below, items are listed according to the media with which they are used. Be sure to purchase everything you need for each activity you expect to include in your clinical repertoire. Some items are used so frequently that they are considered basic and should be in every clinic.

Basic items:

Cardboard
Pencils
Scissors
Craft knife
Rule(r)
Measuring tape
Paper
Newspaper
Kraft paper
Paper towel
Water source
Masking tape
Cellophane tape
Wood glue
White glue
Sponges
Rags

Basketry:

Wooden bases
Reed
Clippers
Fid
Water pail

Spinning:

Fleece
Cards (pair of wire brushes)
Drop spindle
Spinning wheel

Latch hooking:

Canvas
Cut yarn or yarn cutter
Latchet hook

Macramé:

Jute or cord
Brass ring (2 inch)

Knitting:

Yarn
Knitting needles
Tapestry needle

Sewing:

Fabric
Patterns

Chalk
Tracing paper
Tracing wheel
Straight pins
Needles
Thread
Pin cushion
Thimble
Stitch ripper
Assorted buttons
Sewing machine
Stuffing (fiberfill or cut-up nylon stockings)

Embroidery:

Fabric
Floss
Embroidery needles
Embroidery hoop
Thimble

Crewel:

Fabric
Crewel yarn
Tapestry needles
Thimble
Embroidery hoop

Ceramics:

Wedging board or oil cloth
Clay
Elephant ear sponge
Kemper tool
Turntable
Rolling pin
Plaster bat
Wheel
Wire
Plaster molds
Slip
Sandpaper
Glaze

Mosaics:

Base
Tiles
Tile cutter
Cement
Grout
Silicone polish

Leathercrafts:

Leathers
Tooler

Steel rule
Utility shears
Rubber cement
Slit punch
Rotary punch
Single-hole punch
Lacing
Leather needle
Duco cement
Skiver
Stamping tools
Sandpaper
Leather dye
Leather polish
Soft cloth
Awl
Mallet
Tapestry needles
Button thread
Beeswax
Stamping tools

Copper tooling:

Copper foil
Molds
Masking tape
Tooler
Orangewood stick
Metal shears
Liver of sulfur
Steel wool
Wooden plaque
Stain
Varnish
Awl
Hammer
Escutcheon pins
Acrylic spray

Enameling:

Copper blanks
Steel wool
Gum of tragacanth
Enamel
Enameling kiln
Earring and pin backs

Wire jewelry:

Copper wire, 16 or 18 gauge
Needle-nose pliers
Flat-nose pliers
Wire cutter
Steel wool

Woodworking:

Woods
Claw hammer
Phillips head screwdriver
Slit head screwdriver
Cross-cut saw
Table jigsaw
Electric drill
Drill bits, assorted sizes
Clamps
Vise
Half-round file
Rasp
Sandpaper—coarse and fine
Level
Carpenter's square
Chisel
Mallet
Doweling
Wood glue
Stain
Varnish
Rags
Screws
Nails

Wiring:

Threaded metal tube
Bolts
Electric wire
Plug
Lamp socket
Wire stripper

Penny switch:

Copper pennies
Steel wool
Wire
Single-socket plug
Soldering iron
Solder
Flux

Papermaking:

Cotton or linen rags
Fabric dye
Mold and deckle frame
Wooden board
Weight
Food processor
Rectangular pan

Papier Mâché:

Newspaper
Flour

Oil of wintergreen
Balloons
Egg cartons
Plasticene

Greeting cards:

Tissue paper
Food coloring
Plastic containers
Freezer wrap
Electric iron
Roasting pan

Marbled paper:

Paper
Tempera paints
Vegetable oil
Aluminum pan

Block printing:

Paper
Linoleum block
Chisels
Brayer
Ink

Stenciling:

Stencil paper or used x-ray film
Stencil brush
Elephant Ear sponge
X-acto knife
Package of stationery or other blank paper
Tempera paints

Silk screening:

Paper
Silk-screen frame
Stencil paper
X-acto knife
Rubber squeegee
Printing ink
Clothesline
Clothespins
Masking tape

Bookbinding:

White paper
Ornamental paper
Awl
Clamps
Wooden press
Tapestry needle
Button thread
Beeswax
Fabric

Spoon
Spine cloth (organdy)

Photography:

Camera
Film
Batteries

Videotaping:

Camera
Videotapes
Videorecorder
Television set
Cables
Editing equipment (optional)

Computers:

Computer

Keyboard
Mouse
Video screen
Software
Cables
Printer
Surge protector

Adaptive devices for computers and technology:

Joy stick
Light pen
Power pad
Puff-sip device
Speech synthesizer

Telecommunications:

Modem
Fax

APPENDIX C

Commercial Sources of Supply

CRAFTS

American Art Clay Co., Inc. (AMACO)
4717 W. 16th St.
Indianapolis, IN 46222
(317)244-0871
(800)374-1600
(317)248-9300 Fax

Association of People Who Play with Dolls
1779 East Avenue
Hayward, CA 94541

Colophon Book Arts Supply
3046 Hoqum Bay Road NE
Olympia, WA 98516
(206)459-2940

Constantine's
2050 Eastchester Rd.
Bronx, NY 10461
(800)233-8087
Specialty wood items

Craftime, Inc.
PO Box 93706
Atlanta, GA 30377
(404)873-2028
(404)876-6428 Fax
(800)849-8463

Dick Blick Company
PO Box 1267
Galesburg, IL 61401
(309)343-6181 ext. 235
(800)933-2542

Dremel, Inc.
4915 21st Street
Racine, WI 53406
(414)554-1390

Nasco
901 Jamesville Ave.
Ft. Atkinson, WI 53538-0901
(414)563-2446
(414)563-8296 Fax

Paxton/Patterson
1003A Greentree
Executive Campus
Marlton, NJ 08053
(800)631-0158
(609)985-3457 Fax
(609)985-8877 Local

Royal Arts & Crafts
650 Ethel Street NW
Atlanta, GA 30318
(404)881-0075

S & S Worldwide
75 Mill St.
Colchester, CT 06415
(203)537-3451
(203)537-2866 Fax
(800)937-3482 Customer Service

Sax Arts and Crafts
2405 Calhoun Road
PO Box 51710
New Berlin, WI 53151
(414)784-6880

Tandy Leather Company
1400 Everman Parkway
Ft. Worth, TX 76140
(817)551-9781

Triarco Arts and Crafts, Inc.
14650 28th Ave. N.
Plymouth, MI 55447
(612)559-5590

Veteran Leather
204 25th Street
Brooklyn, NY 11232-9970
(718)768-0300
(718)768-8361 Fax

TECHNOLOGY

AbleNet, Inc.
1081 Tenth Ave., SE
Minneapolis, MN 55414
(800)322-0956

Access Unlimited — SPEECH Enterprises
9039 Katy Freeway
Suite 414
Houston, TX 77024
(713)461-0006

adaptAbility
PO Box 515
Colchester, CT 06415-0515
(800)243-9232

Adaptive Communication Systems
354 Hookstown Grade Road
Clinton, PA 15206
(412)264-2288

Arctic Technologies
55 Park St.
Suite 2
Troy, MI 48083
(313)588-7370

Boston Educational Systems & Technology, Inc.
 (B.E.S.T.)
63 Forest Street
Chestnut Hill, MA 02167
(617)277-0179
(617)277-1275 Fax

Boswell Industries, Inc.
Suite 630
470 Granville St.
Vancouver, BC V6C 1V5
Canada
(604)684-3629

Computability Corporation
4000 Grand River
Suite 109
Novi, MN 48375
(313)477-6720

Compute Able Network, Inc.
PO Box 1706
Portland, OR 97207
(503)645-0009
(503)645-2049 Fax

Computerized Enabling System
19 North 8th Street
Kenilworth, NJ 07033
(201)276-6769

Crabapple Systems
124 Gray Road
Falmouth, ME 04105
(207)797-2388

Digital Equipment Corporation
129 Parker Street
Maynard, MA 01754
(800)832-6277
(617)897-5111

DLM Teaching Resources
One DLM Park
Allen, TX 75002
(800)527-5030

Don Johnston Developmental Equipment, Inc.
1000 North Rand Road, Bldg. 115
Wauconda, IL 60084
(800)999-4660

Dragon Systems (voice activated)
320 Nevada Street
Newton, MA 02158
(617)965-5200

Du-It Control Systems Group
8765 Township Road #513
Shreve, OH 44676
(216)567-2001

Dunamis, Inc.
3620 Highway 317
Swanee, GA 30174
(404)932-0485

EKEG Electronics
PO Box 46199
Station D
Vancouver, BC V6J 5G5
Canada
(604)273-4358
(604)273-1418 Fax

Extensions for Independence
757 Emory Street #514
Imperial Beach, CA 92032
(619) 426-8054

Fox Bay Industries (wrist support)
4150 B Place, NW
Kent, WA 98031
(206)941-9155

Fred Sammons, Inc.
PO Box 0697, Dept. 728
Grand Rapids, MI 49501-3697
(800)323-5547

Free Software Foundation (keystroke reduction)
675 Massachusetts Ave.
Cambridge, MA 02139
(617)876-3296

Frog Computer Systems, Inc.
101 Golf Course Drive, Suite A220
Rohnert Park, CA 94928
(707)586-2255

Handicapped Children's Technology
PO Box 7
Foster, RI 02825
(401)861-3444

Health Care Keyboard Company, Inc.
N82 W15340 Appleton Ave.
Menononee Falls, WI 53051
(414)253-4131

Henter-Joyce, Inc.
The Experts in Access Technology
10901-C Roosevelt Blvd.
Suite 1200
St. Petersburg, FL 33716
(813)576-5658
(813)577-0099 Fax
(800)336-5658

Anthony Hodges (V-shaped keyboard)
Mountain View, CA 94040

Kinesis Corporation
915 118 Avenue, SE
Bellevue, WA 98004
(206)455-9220

MicroComputer (Rubbermaid wrist support)
960 N. San Antonio Road
Los Altos, CA
(415)941-6679

North Coast Medical (wrist support)
187 Stouffer Boulevard
San Jose, CA
(408)283-1900

Silicon Sports (wrist support)
324 High Street
Palo Alto, CA
(415)327-7900

Michale J. Soucha
East Wind Community
RT3 Box 6B2
Tecumseh, MO 65760
(417)679-4682

Regenesis Development Corporation
4381 Galant Ave.
North Vancouver, BC V7G 1L1
(604)929-2414

RESNA
1101 Connecticut Avenue, NW
Suite 700
Washington, DC 20036
(202)857-1199

Sentient Systems Tech, Inc.
5001 Baum Blvd.
Pittsburgh, PA 15213
(412)682-0144

TASH, Inc.
91 Station St.
Unit 1
Ajax, ON LIS 3H2
Canada
(905)686-4129

Tangent Designs, Inc.
3954 NE 115th St.
Seattle, WA 98125
(206)367-5826
Mobile arm support for computer keyboard

Trace Research & Development Center
S-151 Waisman Center
1500 Highland Avenue
Madison, WI 53705
(608)262-6966

Unicorn Engineering, Inc.
5221 Central Ave.
Suite 205
Richmond, CA 94804
(415)528-0670

TeleSensory
455 North Bernardo Ave.
Mountain View, CA 94043
(415)960-0920
(800)227-8418

Venture Technologies, Inc.
304 134 Abbott Street
Vancouver, BC V6B 2K4
Canada
(604)684-9803

Votrax Corporation
1358 Rankin
Troy, MI 48083
Speech synthesizer

Worldwide Disabilities Solutions Group
Apple Computer
20525 Mariani Ave. MS36SE
Cupertino, CA 95014
(408)974-7910

Zygo Industries, Inc.
PO Box 1008
Portland, OR 97207-1008
(503)684-6006

SOFTWARE

Arctic Technologies
55 Park St.
Suite 2
Troy, MI 48083
(313)588-7370

Boston Educational Systems & Technology, Inc.
  (B.E.S.T.)
63 Forest Street
Chestnut Hill, MA 02167
(617)277-0179
(617)277-1275 Fax

Braintree, Inc.
1915 Huguenot Road
Richmond, VA 23235
(804)794-4841
(800)633-1221 Fax
(800)794-3916 Fax

Broderbund Software, Inc.
500 Redwood Blvd.
PO Box 6121
Novato, CA 94948-6121
(415)382-4400

Brown Bag Software
2155 South Bascom
Suite 114
Campbell, CA 95008
(408)559-4545

Bucks County Intermediate
Unit #22
705 Shady Retreat
Doylestown, PA 18902
(215)348-2940 ext. 361

Cambridge Development Laboratory, Inc.
1696 Massachusetts Ave.
Cambridge, MA 02138
(800)637-0047
(617)491-0377 in MA

Captain's Log
Braintrain
727 Twin Ridge La.
Richmond, VA 23235
(804)320-0105
(804)320-0242 Fax

Center for Adapted Technology (shareware)
Colorado Easter Seal Society
5775 W. Almeda Ave.
Lakewood, CO 80226
(303)233-1666

COMPUSERVE
PO Box 20212
5000 Arlington Center Blvd.
Columbus, OH 43220
(800)848-8199

Computability
101 Route 46 East
Pine Brook, NJ 07058
(908)882-0171

Computer Conversations
2350 North Fourth St.
Columbus, OH 43202
(614)263-4324
Talking word processing program

CREATE
Theodore I. King, II
PO Box 28
Hales Corners, WI 53130
(414)529-4964

CREATE: Cognitive Rehabilitation Evaluation and
  Treatment Exercises
Phyllis Criter
PO Box 8896
Green Bay, WI 54308

Cursor Program, Public Domain Software
High Tech Center
Chancellor's Office
1107 Ninth Street
Sacramento, CA 95814
(916)322-4636

Don Johnston Developmental Equipment Corp.
1000 N. Rand Road #115
PO Box 639
Wauconda, IL 60084
(708)526-2682

DSH (Discount Software House)
PO Box 93
Winnebago, WI 54985
(800)543-3277 orders only
(414)231-1696 customer service

Dunamis, Inc.
3620 Highway 317
Swanee, GA 30174
(404)932-0485

Easter Seal and Lehigh Valley Computer Project
    (shareware)
PO Box 333
Kulpsville, PA 19443
(215)368-7000

Educational Electronics Co. Ltd.
PO Box 46199
Station G
Vancouver, BC V6R 4G5
(604)273-4358
(604)273-1148 Fax

ETHOM ASSOCIATES
4595 Club Drive
Atlanta, GA 30319
(404)237-3851

Exceptional Children's Software, Inc.
PO Box 4758
Overland Park, KS 66204
(913)831-3800

FPCL Software
PO Box 160999
Altamonte Springs, FL 32716

Fred Sammons, Inc.
PO Box 0697, Dept. 728
Grand Rapids, MI 49501-3697
(800)323-5547

Handicapped Children's Technology
PO Box 7
Foster, RI 02825
(401)861-3444

Hartley Courseware, Inc.
Coolidge Road
Dimondale, MI 48821
(517)646-6458 in Michigan
(800)247-1380
(517)646-8451 Fax

Laureate Learning Systems
110 East Spring St.
Winooski, VT 05404
(802)655-4755

Qualitative Research Management
73-425 Hilltop Road
Desert Hot Springs, CA 92240
(619)329-7026

Psychological Software Services
6555 Carrollton Ave.
Indianapolis, IN 46220
(317)257-9672

R.J. Cooper & Associates (shareware)
Adaptive Technology Specialists
24843 Del Prado #283
Dana Point, CA 92629
(714)240-1912

Special Education Software Center
Building B. Room S312
333 Ravenswood Ave.
Menlo Park, CA 94025
(800)327-5892

Spies Laboratories
4040 Spencer St.
Suite Q
Torrence, CA 90503
(213)538-8166
Enlarged test on print out

Spinnaker Software Corporation
201 Broadway
Cambridge, MA 02139
(617)494-1200

Sunburst Communications
39 Washington Avenue
Pleasantville, NY 10570-2898
(800)431-1934

Teachers' Institute for Special Education, Inc.
2947 Bayside Court
Wantagh, NY 11793
(516)781-2020

Technology for Language and Learning (shareware)
Catalogue of Public Domain Software
PO Box 327
East Rockaway, NY 11518-0327
(516)625-4550

UCLA Intervention Program for Handicapped Children
1000 Veteran Ave. Room 23-10
Los Angeles, CA 90024
(310)825-4321

World Communications
245 Tonopah Drive
Fremont, CA 94539
(415)656-0911

The Activity Analysis Form

ACTIVITY ANALYSIS

Activity: _____

Student: _____

Date: _____

EGOCENTRIC ELEMENTS

(all aspects of mind and body)

MIND

Numerous theorists, Piaget, Freud, Maslow, Erikson, and Gilligan among them, have described ways in which the mind develops. These include the development of learning, emotion, and social awareness. The following are various aspects of the mind.

PERCEPTION

Self-Image (identity):

Body Image:

Discrimination:

of self from other person(s):

of self from other object(s):

---

of body parts from each other (gnosis):

---

of objects from one another (stereognosis):

Figure-Ground:

Form Constancy:

Spatial Orientation (e.g., vertical, horizontal, diagonal):

Laterality (sidedness of self):

Directionality (way finding):

Memory (recognition):

Symbolism:

COGNITION (deliberate, focused attention)

Problem Solving:

Doubt (wonder):

Inquiry:

Intellect:

Learning:

Memory (recall):

MOTIVATION

Internal Direction (innate drives, e.g., hunger eliciting eating):

Volition/Will (learned intention, e.g., eating as a plan to avoid hunger):

AFFECT/EMOTION

Happiness:

_____

Sadness:

_____

Anger:

_____

DYNAMIC STATES

Alertness:

_____

Frustration Tolerance:

_____

Self-Control:

_____

Reality Testing:

Gratification:

Immediate:

Delayed:

TEMPORALITY (subjective)

Immediate:

Distant:

Speed:

Sequence:

Present:

Past:

Future:

SPIRITUALITY

Religion:

Ethics/Morality:

BODY

Many aspects of the body are essential to activity. Some of these are evident at birth, some are developed according to a predetermined schedule, some are acquired by experience and practice. These components all interact.

PHYSIOLOGICAL

Cardiovascular:

Respiratory:

Toxicity:

Immunological:

Allergic:

Skin Integrity:

_____

Biorhythms:

_____

MOTOR COMPONENTS

Reflexes and Reactions:

Stretch:

_____

Blink:

_____

Sneeze:

_____

Balance:

_____

Equilibrium Reactions:

Nystagmus:

Orgasm:

Posture and Position:

Prone:

Supine:

Side-Lying:

Quadruped:

Sitting:

Standing:

DEVELOPMENTAL READINESS:

All items below are necessary precursors to movement patterns in adults and the activities in which they

engage.

Head Turning:

Tracking:

Righting Reactions:

Rolling:

Creeping:

Crawling:

Sitting:

Grasp:

Standing:

Walking:

_____

Climbing:

_____

Running:

_____

Speaking:

_____

Jumping:

_____

Hopping:

_____

Skipping:

_____

RANGE OF MOTION

Head/Neck:

Trunk:

Limbs:

Upper Extremities:

Lower Extremities:

MUSCLE POWER

Head/Neck:

Trunk:

Limbs:

   Upper Extremities:

   Lower Extremities:

   Endurance:

COORDINATION:

   Head/Neck:

   Trunk:

Limbs:

Upper Extremities:

_____

Unilateral:

_____

Bilateral:

_____

Symmetrical:

_____

Asymmetrical:

_____

Lower Extremities:

Unilateral:

_____

Bilateral:

Symmetrical:

Asymmetrical:

Upper and Lower Extremities:

Symmetrical:

Asymmetrical:

Grasp:

Cylindrical:

Spherical:

_____

Hook:

_____

Lateral Pinch:

_____

3-Jaw Chuck:

_____

Fingertip Pinch:

_____

Hand/Arm:

_____

Fingers:

SENSORY COMPONENTS

Near Sensors:

Taste (e.g., sweet, sour, bitter, salty):

Touch:

Light Touch:

Deep Touch:

Temperature:

Pain:

_____

Vibration:

_____

Proprioception (movement of body parts):

_____

Vestibular:

    Movement of Head:

_____

    Movement through Space:

_____

Kinesthesia (integration of proprioceptive and vestibular inputs):

_____

Distance Sensors:

Smell:

Scent Recognition:

Directionality:

Vision:

Monocular:

Binocular:

Color:

Contrast:

Distance:

Near (accommodation):

_____

Far:

_____

Foveal:

_____

Peripheral:

_____

Ambient:

_____

Static:

_____

Moving:

    Object:

    Self:

Hearing:

    Monaural:

    Dichodic:

    Volume:

Discriminant (auditory figure ground):

> **EXOCENTRIC ELEMENTS (all aspects of external**
>
> **space/time and tangible objects**
>
> **also known as the nonhuman environment and temporal**
>
> **dimension)**

OBJECTS (manipulable)

  Food:

  _____

  Toys:

  _____

  Tools:

  _____

  Materials:

  _____

  Equipment:

Furniture:

SPATIAL ENVIRONMENT (ordinarily beyond the limits of manipulation)

Space:

Terrain:

Weather:

Time Zone:

TEMPORAL ENVIRONMENT

Past:

Present:

_____

Future:

_____

Speed:

_____

Duration:

_____

Delays:

_____

Rhythm:

_____

CONSENSUAL ELEMENTS

(all aspects of relationships or communication with

others)

DYADIC RELATIONSHIPS

Parent/Child:

Spousal:

Friendships:

Employer/Employee:

Coworker:

SMALL GROUP RELATIONSHIPS

Family:

_____

Friends:

_____

Peers:

_____

Coworkers:

_____

Teams:

_____

SOCIAL INTERACTIONS

Communication:

_____

Cooperation:

Competition:

Negotiation:

Assertiveness:

Compromise:

SOCIAL RESPONSIBILITY

Caring:

For Self:

For Others:

Play:

School:

Work:

SOCIETAL INFLUENCES

Ethnicity:

Customs:

Rules:

___

Gender Roles:

___

Peer Pressure:

___

Economics:

___

Education:

___

APPENDIX E

Bibliography

Addams, J: Twenty Years at Hull House. Macmillan, New York, 1910.

Addams, J: My Friend Julia Lathrop. Ayer, Salem, NH, 1935.

Am Occup Ther Assoc: Resolution 531. AOTA, Rockville, MD, April 1979.

Auel, J: Clan of the Cave Bear. Bantam, New York, 1980.

Auel, J: Valley of the Horses. Bantam, New York, 1983.

Auel, J: Mammoth Hunters. Bantam, New York, 1986.

Auel, J: Plains of Passage. Bantam, New York, 1989.

Ayres, AJ: Sensory Integration and Learning Theory. Western Psychological Services, Los Angeles, 1972.

Bandura, A: Psychological Modeling: Conflicting Theories. Aldine-Atherton, Chicago, 1971.

Bing, RK: William Rush Dunton, Jr. American psychiatrist: A study in self. EdD dissertation, University of Maryland, 1961.

Bing, RK: Eleanor Clarke Slagle lectureship: Occupational therapy revisited: A paraphrastic journey. Am J Occup Ther 35:499–518, 1981.

Breines, EB: Perception: Its Development and Recapitulation. Geri-Rehab, Lebanon, NJ, 1981.

Breines, EB: An attempt to define purposeful activity. Am J Occup Ther 38:543–544, 1984.

Breines, EB: Origins and Adaptations: A Philosophy of Practice. Geri-Rehab, Lebanon, NJ, 1986.

Breines, EB: Making a difference: Implications for education and health. Am J Occup Ther 43:40–41, 1989.

Breines, EB: Media education based on the philosophy of pragmatism. Am J Occup Ther 43:461–464, 1989.

Breines, EB: Emil G. Hirsch: Pioneer figure in occupational therapy. Judaism 38:216–223, 1989.

Breines, EB: Genesis of occupation: A philosophical model for therapy. Australian Occup Ther J 37:45–49, 1990.

Breines, EB: Rabbi Emil G. Hirsch: Ethical philosopher and founding figure of occupational therapy. Israel J Occup Ther 1:1–10, 1992.

Cohen, S: The mental hygiene movement. The development of personality and the school: The medicalization of American education. History of Education Quarterly 23:123–149, 1983.

Craft Techniques in Occupational Therapy, Department of the Army, Washington, DC, 1980.

Cynkin, S: Occupational Therapy: Toward Health Through Activities. Little, Brown, Boston. 1979.

Darwin, CR: The Origin of Species by Means of Natural Selection. Macmillan-Collier, New York, 1859.

Dewey, J: Democracy and Education: An Introduction to the Philosophy of Education. Collier-Macmillan, Toronto, 1916.

Dewey, J: The Quest for Certainty: A Study of the Relation of Knowledge and Action. Minton, Balch, New York, 1929.

Dunton, WR: Occupation Therapy: A Manual for Nurses. WB Saunders, Philadelphia, 1915.

Edgerton, SG: Independence through sharing: The vocational planning of Heinrich Pestalozzi — renowned Swiss educator. History of Education Quarterly 14:403–406, 1974.

English, C, Karsch, H, Silverman, P, and Walker, S: On the role of occupational therapists in physical disabilities. Am J Occup Ther 36:199–202, 1982.

Erikson, E: Childhood and Society. WW Norton, New York, 1986.

Fidler, GS: Professional or nonprofessional. In Occupational Therapy 2001. American Occupational Therapy Association, Rockville, Maryland, 1979.

Fidler, GS: From crafts to competence. Am J Occup Ther 35:567–573, 1981.

Fidler, GS and Fidler, JW: Doing and becoming: Purposeful action and self-actualization. Am J Occup Ther 32:305–310, 1978.

Freud, S: General Psychological Theory. Collier, New York, 1963.

Freud, S: Totem and Taboo. Random House, New York, 1918, 1946.

Gibson, JJ: The Senses Considered as Perceptual Systems. Houghton Mifflin, Boston, 1966.

Gilligan, C: In a Different Voice: Psychological Theory and Women's Development. Harvard University Press, Cambridge, MA, 1982.

Gruber, H and Voneche, JJ: The Essential Piaget. Basic Books, New York, 1982.

Hirsch, EG: Laureate oration delivered at the commencement exercises of the Hebrew Union College, Friday evening, June 24, 1892. In Proceeding of the Union of American Hebrew Congregations 4:2951–2963, 1891–1897. American Jewish Archives, Cincinnati Campus, Hebrew Union College, Jewish Institute of Religion.

Hopkins, H and Smith, H (eds): Willard and Spackman's Occupational Therapy, ed 8. Lippincott, Philadelphia, 1993.

Huss, AJ: From kinesiology to adaptation. Am J Occup Ther 35:574, 1981.

Keller, E: A Feeling for the Organism: The Life and Work of Barbara McClintock. WH Freeman, New York, 1983.

Koestler, A: Insight and Outlook: An Inquiry into the Common Foundations of Science, Art and Social Ethics. Macmillan, New York, 1949.

Leakey, R and Lewin, R: Origins Reconsidered: In Search of What Makes Us Human. Doubleday, New York, 1992.

Levine, R: The influence of the Arts-and-Crafts movement on the professional status of occupational therapy. Am J Occup Ther 41:248–254, 1987.

Levinson, RE: Mind at Large: Knowing in the Technological Age. JAI, Greenwich, CT, 1988.

Loebl, D: Creative Uses for Computers in Special Education and Cognitive Rehabilitation. Pelican, Fairfield, CT, 1991.

Marshall, EM: Occupational Therapy: Fundamentals of Work. Slack, Thorofare, NJ, 1975.

Maslow, A: Psychology of Science: A Reconnaissance. Regnary Gateway, Washington, DC, 1966.

Mayhew, KC and Edwards, AC: The Dewey School: The Lab School of the University of Chicago, 1896–1903. Appleton-Century, New York, 1936.

Mead, GH: Philosophy of the Present. Murphy, AE (ed). Open Court, Chicago, 1932.

Mead, GH: The Philosophy of the Act. University of Chicago Press, Chicago, 1938.

Meyer, A: The Collected Papers of Adolf Meyer. In EE Winters (ed). Johns Hopkins Press, Baltimore, 1952.

Meyer, A: The philosophy of occupation therapy. Arch Occup Ther 1:1–10, 1922.

Peloquin, SM: Occupational therapy service: Individual and collective understandings of the founders, Part 1. Am J Occup Ther 45:352–363, 1991.

Peloquin, SM: Occupational therapy service: Individual and collective understandings of the founders, Part 2. Am J Occup Ther 45:733–744, 1991.

Penrose, R: The Emperor's New Mind: Concerning Computers, Minds and the Laws of Physics. Oxford, New York, 1989.

Piaget, J: Behavior and Evolution. D. Nicholson-Smith, trans. Pantheon, New York, 1978.

Reed, KL: Eleanor Clarke Slagle lecture. Tools of practice: Heritage or baggage? Am J Occup Ther 40:597–605, 1986.

Reilly, M: Play as Exploratory Learning. Sage, Beverly Hills, CA, 1974.

Slagle, EC: Training aides for mental patients. Arch Occup Ther 1:11–17, 1922.

Smith, J: The Idea of Health: Implications for the Nursing Professional. Columbia University Press, New York, 1983.

Smith, RO, Hammel, J, Rein, J, and Anson, D: Technology as an occupational therapy treatment modality. OT Week, March 5, 1992.

Tracy, SE: Studies in Invalid Occupations: A Manual for Nurses and Attendants. Whitcomb and Barrows, Boston, 1918.

Trombly, CA: Include exercise in "purposeful activity." Am J Occup Ther 36:467–468, 1982.

von Bertalannfy, L: General Systems Theory. George Braziller, New York, 1962.

Welker, WI: An analysis of exploratory and play behavior in animals. In Fiske, DW and Maddi, SR (eds): Functions of Varied Experience. Dorsey, Homewood, IL, 1961, pp 175–226.

Washburn, SL: Tools and human evolution. Sci Am 203:1960.

White, RN: Ego and Reality in Psychoanalytic Theory. In Psychological Issues 3: International Universities Press, New York, 1959.

White, RN: Motivation reconsidered: The concept of competence. In Fiske, DW and Maddi, SR (eds): Functions of Varied Experience. Dorsey, Homewood, IL, (1961) pp 278–325.

Index

Numbers followed by an "f" indicate figures; numbers followed by a "t" indicate tables.